Living in Hope

A 12-Step Approach for
Persons at Risk or Infected with HIV

CINDY MIKLUSCAK-COOPER, R.N.
& EMMETT E. MILLER, M.D.

CELESTIAL ARTS
Berkeley, California

ACKNOWLEDGEMENT

We would like to thank all the brave and selfless people who shared their experience, strength and hope with us in order to help those who follow. The generosity of all the Carls, Louises and Ryans and those who remain nameless is deeply appreciated and honored. You live on in our hearts and in these pages.

The Twelve Steps of Alcoholics Anonymous have been reprinted and adapted with the permission of A.A. World Services, Inc., New York, NY 10163

Quotations from *Alcoholics Anonymous* (copyright 1939, 1955, 1976), *Twelve Steps and Twelve Traditions* (copyright 1952, 1953) and *As Bill Sees It* (copyright 1967) by Alcoholics Anonymous World Services, Inc. reprinted with their permission.

Quotations from *Touch of Silence* (copyright 1989) by Cosmoenergetics Publications reprinted with author, Jan Kennedy's permission.

Cover and text design by Nancy Austin
Composition by Pamela Meyer
Photo of C. Mikluscak-Cooper by Connie Stone

FIRST PRINTING, 1991

Library of Congress Cataloging-in-Publication Data

Mikluscak-Cooper, Cindy, 1947–
   Living in hope: a 12 step approach for persons at risk or
infected with HIV / Cindy Mikluscak-Cooper and Emmett Miller.
    p.   cm.
Includes bibliographical references.
ISBN 0-89087-629-0
   1. AIDS (Disease)—Psychological aspects. 2. Twelve-step
programs. I. Miller, Emmett E. II. Title.
RC607.A26M54   1991
616.97'92—dc20
                                             90-2611
                                             CIP

1   2   3   4   5   6   7   8   9   0   /   95   94   93   92   91

CONTENTS

DEDICATION

This book is dedicated to the men, women and children who have been affected by the disease known as AIDS. Your courage and humanity serve as an eternal guiding light for all who suffer in their own birthing, living and dying. We are forever grateful.

INTRODUCTION

Where There's Hope, There's Life

From the beginning of the AIDS (Acquired Immune Deficiency Syndrome) epidemic, we have been deeply moved by the pain and suffering of our patients, friends, and colleagues. At first little was available to help people deal with this unprecedented challenge. Through more than two decades of personal work and healing we have acquired some powerful tools that have proven valuable to us and to millions of people attempting to cope with all sorts of life-threatening illnesses. This book, the result of more than six years of intensive research and loving attention to the AIDS dilemma, is about these tools. It describes, step by step, how these life-enhancing skills can be helpful to those affected by this tragedy.

In some way your life has been dramatically affected by AIDS. You probably have a yearning in your heart and anxious questions in your mind. We believe that, as Norman Cousins said, "The tragedy of life is not death, but what we let die inside us while we live." We hope you find solace, courage, and gentle guidance in the perspectives and suggestions here. We offer them to assist you in keeping alive that spirit within that gives life its true value.

The Changing Face of HIV Infection

Our outlook on AIDS and infection caused by HIV, is very different from that of a few years ago. In early 1991, the *average* time from infection to the onset of AIDS was believed to be eleven years. HIV infection and AIDS are *not* synonymous. AIDS is just one end of the spectrum of HIV infection. With early treatment intervention, the number of people who do *not* progress to AIDS can be significantly higher. HIV infection is no longer a death sentence!

At the 1989 National AIDS Update, Marcus Conant, M.D., of the California State Task Force on AIDS, stated, "Hope fulfills itself—hope begets hope, and there is now reason to hope." And from our experience, as well as that of our colleagues, patients, and friends, we know that the twelve-step program developed by Alcoholics Anonymous, and other techniques, such as behavior modification, thought restructuring, positive self-talk, imagery, and other active coping skills, can empower you with this life-sustaining hope. You *can* improve your life emotionally, mentally, spiritually, and physically. Where there is hope, there *is* life—and today there *is* hope.

As you read this book it will become obvious that everyone could benefit from these tools. But when confronted with a crisis, such as an addiction or HIV infection, life seems more precious. You naturally yearn to live life to its fullest. It is this desire that often leads to the exploration of new ways of being, such as those embodied in twelve-step programs and the other techniques offered here.

This program is *not* intended as a cure or a guarantee of recovery, but it *is* a path that can improve your chances for a more fulfilling and longer life.

How Can this Book Help You?

- *If you are infected or have any HIV-related conditions or AIDS,* this program teaches you specific skills for dealing with your emotional, mental, and spiritual needs. Learning these skills can affect your physical symptoms. This program also describes what to avoid to prevent further illness and what to strive for to optimize your health.

- *If you are concerned but unclear as to your infection status,* you can learn how to better manage that uncertainty.

- *If you are worried about becoming infected,* this book shows you how best to avoid infection.

- *If you are suffering from "survivor guilt,"* you can develop new tools for working through this guilt and moving on to a more peaceful acceptance of your life and yourself.

- *If you are in a relationship with someone who is at risk of developing or infected with HIV,* you can learn how to help and nurture yourself, your friend, and your relationship.

- *If you lack a spiritual source of strength*, this program presents a nonreligious model of spirituality that has helped millions throughout the world. With it you can discover your own spiritual reservoir of hope and comfort.

- *If you are a helping professional*, this book expands your knowledge about HIV infection, addictions, abuse issues, and twelve-step programs. It also adds to your understanding of the pain, loneliness, isolation, and depression with which your clients may struggle.

In confronting the many aspects of HIV infection, you may feel some strong, paralyzing emotions. You may be scared because the future is so much less certain than it once seemed. You may feel devastated by the loss of friends and acquaintances. You may be grieving or still in shock because of all you have lost or fear you may lose. You may feel cheated and abused.

You are probably furious. You may find yourself experiencing prolonged depressions or mood swings and may be using alcohol, drugs, or other means of attempting to escape the pain. Or you may have worked through many of these intense feelings, yet on occasion may experience a returning sense of impending doom.

If you are infected, and especially if you have symptoms of AIDS, your emotions may feel overwhelming at times. Perhaps you've cried, screamed, kicked, and thrown things—or become numb, seemingly suspended in space and time. You may have become obsessed with your physical symptoms. Perhaps you've desperately searched for a cure or for someone who has answers. Maybe you've even felt like giving up: "Why even bother! Nothing I do makes any difference anyhow!"

You have every right to be outraged.

And it's normal to have fantasies of giving up. That's part of coping with the shock, as are the overwhelming emotions. You may *feel* hopeless and helpless. But this situation is *not* hopeless.

You are *not* helpless. You have choices and your choices *can* make a difference. We want to help you identify these choices. How you deal with this crisis, how you handle your behaviors and feelings, may have a dramatic impact on the quality and length of your life.

Why a Twelve-Step Approach?

Owing to the unprecedented success of Alcoholics Anonymous (AA) in helping alcoholics and other chemically dependent people for more than fifty years, many other groups have successfully adapted its basic framework, the twelve steps. These same twelve steps can help people at risk of developing or infected with HIV deal with the denial, the anxiety, the shame, the anger and depression, the fear and the loneliness, as well as other feelings that arise.

HIV infection and AIDS have much in common with alcoholism and drug addiction. Like alcoholism, HIV infection is poorly understood by most of society and is often seen as a moral issue rather than a physical disease. This same lack of understanding and fear leads to social rejection; sometimes even a person's friends and family back away. Feelings of shame and guilt are seen with both conditions. HIV infection, like alcoholism, has an insidious onset, has no clear cure, and is a chronic condition that can lead to premature death.

HIV infection and alcoholism share another dangerous quality: denial. Many people who abuse alcohol or drugs, as well as the people close to them, would rather not think about or deal with the addiction. Frequently this is the case with people infected with HIV. It is as if avoiding the topic or referring to "it" only jokingly will make "it" go away. The problem is that it won't go away. All denial does is prevent diagnosis and interfere with treatment. Denial hinders the development of coping strategies, thus making a troubling situation even worse.

A sense of self-esteem and competence is crucial for developing and maintaining the long-term behavior changes necessary for chronic conditions. The HIV-infected person or person at risk needs support and guidance in dealing with behavior change as well as losses, tangible and intangible. Self-hatred and shame can keep him or her feeling alienated, depressed, even self-destructive. The "one day at a time" philosophy of AA enables people to deal

4

with these issues and maintain prolonged sobriety while promoting competence. A large percentage of those with HIV infection abuse alcohol or drugs. A twelve-step approach can be especially helpful to them and to anyone dealing with his or her own or another's HIV infection or risk of infection.

The essence of the AA approach is, "Trouble accepted, trouble squarely faced with calm courage, trouble lessened and often transcended." (Bill Wilson, *As Bill Sees It,* p. 110). This simple method, living on the "twenty-four hour plan," makes for an attitude that fosters health in all dimensions.

Spirit in Action

You can learn, as the millions of recovering alcoholics and addicts have learned, how to tap into that part of yourself that is always healthy, always strong, and always available to you. Many people are able to go beyond the need for physical health in determining their sense of feeling healed: their sense of feeling whole and at peace with themselves and others. They are able to do this by becoming more identified with the spiritual side of themselves, which has no physical limitations. When you nurture and develop yourself spiritually, you can more easily develop emotional states, attitudes, and behaviors that foster health and promote healing. You may be in a very difficult situation, but you can use this tragedy as a chance to awaken: to open to people and to life in a new way and to break any unhealthy habits.

As with other chronic diseases, people with HIV infection, AIDS, or any of the conditions in between often have to deal with numerous changes, including losses. But there are those who survive and even grow through such hardships. Clearly they must be basing their lives on something else, something transcendent.

We often speak of the Higher Power and the spirit. Your spirit plays a vital role in determining whether you feel like a success or a failure, happy or sad, fulfilled or empty. In addition, it plays an important role in health and disease.

A deep sense of meaning is one aspect of spirituality. Viktor Frankl, a psychiatrist, addresses this in his book *Man's Search for Meaning.* He spent three years as an inmate in Nazi concentration camps and sought to answer the question: Why did some die quickly in the camps while others survived the starvation, disease, and cruel conditions?

His answer is that those who survived were those who had some *meaning* in their lives that went beyond the day-to-day suffering. The presence of something to look forward to, even if it was only the eating of a hidden crust of bread, gave them the ability to endure.

Our message includes this spiritual level. We offer you insights and perspectives that you can try out in your own life; tools to gently help you find more meaning and to awaken your own personal spirituality. Those that seem valuable, keep with you and use. Those that do not, set aside and perhaps reexamine later. They may make more sense or be more effective for you then.

What People Alive and Well with HIV Infection and AIDS Tell Us

We interviewed and listened to many people in researching this book. Our goal was to find out what changes in attitude and health behaviors were common to those who were living long and living well with HIV infection or AIDS. Surprisingly, we found great variation in how they managed their disease. Some used only traditional methods, others only nontraditional ones. Most used a combination of both. No specific diets or treatments stood out. What *did* stand out was the assertive way in which they responded to their situation, the vitality of their spirit, and their sense of responsibility for their health and their lives. They attempted to heal their relationships with themselves and others on a daily basis. In seeking enhanced quality, attempting to live each day to the fullest, many were pleasantly surprised to find that the length of their lives was also often enhanced.

Dan T. (in the spirit of the AA principle of anonymity we have chosen not to use full names), who is believed to have acquired HIV infection before or in the early 1980s, was diagnosed with Kaposi's sarcoma in 1981, even before AIDS was a recognized disease. In 1989 he was pursuing a counseling career. When he found out he had AIDS, Dan promised himself he would not let it ruin his life. He assertively sought both traditional medical care as well as alternative therapies, such as acupuncture.

Dan tells us that balance is the key, and that his spiritual and emotional health are a very important part of his recovery. He believes you cannot be healthy if you are at war with yourself or anyone or anything else. "I'm not obsessed with killing off every single cell of the AIDS virus in my body: it would cause me too much stress. We can peacefully cohabit in the same body. If the virus makes me sick again I may have to do something different, but right now I feel pretty good."

His message includes, "Take responsibility for yourself. Find out if you are infected, and then take advantage of everything that is available to help you. Do the things you need to do to stay healthy, and avoid the things you know can harm you. Then live one day at a time, staying as positive and active as possible. Yes, there is life after HIV infection and AIDS!"

Dan's words are remarkably similar to those of the dozen or so long-term AIDS survivors with whom we talked. As defined by the Centers for Disease Control, a long-term survivor (LTS) is someone who has had a diagnosis of full-blown AIDS for more than four years. Many of their thoughts and ideas have been included in this book.

Attitudes and Disease Outcome

Current data strongly suggest that people who succeed in preventing illness or surviving illness longer have certain characteristics and employ similar approaches. These include the many things Dan did, such as using active coping skills, seeking support, and mentally transforming the meaning of events so that they were less stressful. For many years researchers in the field of behavioral medicine have examined how emotional and mental patterns affect outcome in chronic and life-threatening diseases. Recently, several popular and easy to read books have described such studies and suggested methods for maintaining maximum health. These are useful adjuncts to this book. (See Resources appendix.)

In his paper entitled "Mental Adjustment to Cancer as a Factor of Survival" (presented at the conference Current Concepts in Psycho-Oncology and AIDS, held at the Memorial Sloan Kettering Cancer Center in 1987), Steven Greer, M.D., reported that in certain types of cancer, "Patients who survived longer than expected had very positive attitudes towards life and the future, closer personal relationships and coped better with illness-related problems." In addition, "attitudes of stoic acceptance" or "helplessness/hopelessness" were the *least* helpful, and were found in patients who did not survive as long as others. Such findings are consistent with our observations of HIV-infected individuals as well as the observations of others, including Michael Callen of the New York People with AIDS Coalition. Michael Callen edited the informative book *Surviving and Thriving with AIDS: Hints for the Newly Diagnosed* (see Resources appendix). Evidence presented at the Fifth International Conference on AIDS in Montreal, Canada, in 1989, suggests that assertive ways of responding to stress, exercising, using positive imagery, and participating in support groups may affect HIV infection and AIDS. The methods presented in this book address all these areas.

One strategy of coping with illness is to develop a sense of control by learning ways in which you can make a difference. In a classic experiment two rats were placed in identical cages, and both were shocked at the same random times. The rat in cage A learned to stop the shock by pressing a lever. The rat in cage B had no such lever. The immune system of the rat with a control lever was found to remain much stronger than the rat without a lever, despite the fact that they received identical shocks. Other studies have shown that such learned helplessness may affect the human immune system as well. The tools found in a twelve-step program can serve as your control levers. They can help you escape stoic acceptance or helpless/hopeless feelings and assist you in developing ways to take charge.

It is essential to keep in mind, though, that *mental attitude is only one piece of a very big puzzle.* Especially in the case of human disease, scientific studies relating attitudinal and behavioral factors to illness are very difficult to design and analyze, and are not yet conclusive. Many genetic, physical, and environmental factors, as well as behavioral and social ones, influence the course of any infection or disease. It is essential to avoid criticizing yourself or others about the rate of progression of illness. In any specific case other factors might be so predominant that even a dramatic change in attitude and behavior might not significantly alter the course.

But even if the disease cannot be slowed down, living life in a fulfilling fashion, feeling good about yourself, and leaving your body in a peaceful way are worthwhile goals for all of us. How you think and how you feel are extremely important. They determine how you live as well as how you die. At the 1989 National AIDS Update, Dr. Conant reminded us that many HIV-infected individuals told him that the last six months of their lives were better than the rest of their lives had been. Clearly they had found the silver linings within their dark clouds of AIDS.

From Outlook to Outcome: The Mind-Body Link

The body really seems to respond when you send it messages to live. We know this because scientists have the newfound ability to detect chemicals produced by the cells of the nervous and immune systems. The brain and the immune system turn out to be in constant communication with each other through nerve pathways as well as chemical messengers. Neurotransmitters, chemicals produced by the brain, can direct immune cells to mobilize, multiply, and attack harmful invaders.

These chemicals, called "molecules of emotion" by former NIH researcher Candice Pert, Ph.D. are found in high concentration in the feelings and drives center of the brain. This is one way attitudes and expectations can make a difference in the course of infectious disease and cancer. In addition, how we think and feel affects how we act and how we take care of ourselves. Our challenge is to learn to think, act, and express our feelings in ways that foster messages to live.

Keeping the infection under control and your body in good shape until a cure is found is a very reasonable goal. Today the significance of certain co-infections are being realized and successfully managed. New treatments for AIDS and the many aspects of HIV infection are being developed.

The Role of Cofactors

HIV infection can make your body vulnerable to opportunistic infections and cancers. Once any of these develop, the condition is called AIDS. Many people who became infected with HIV have gone on to develop AIDS and then die of complications. But many have not. Luc Montagnier of the Pasteur Institute of Paris, codiscoverer of HIV, says, "AIDS does not inevitably lead to death, especially if you suppress the cofactors that support the disease. . . . Psychological factors are critical in supporting immune function. It simply isn't true that the virus is one hundred percent fatal."

Researchers from The Centers for Disease Control in Atlanta describe men who have been HIV infected for an average of eight years who are well and have *no signs or symptoms of immune system disease*. The HIV appears to be totally inactive. The researchers call these well, yet infected, men *nonprogressors*.

Good health and resistance to disease are the result of many circumstances called cofactors. These include the strength of the immune system, the presence of other infections, the stage of the disease at the time of diagnosis, age, nutrition, sleep, stress responses, freedom from toxins such as drugs and alcohol, exercise, relationships, self-image, emotional balance, and spiritual outlook.

Although you have no direct power over the virus itself, you can change how it affects you by attending to your cofactors. For example, studies repeatedly indicate that alcohol and recreational drugs have negative effects on the immune system and increase the likelihood of high-risk behaviors. These place a person in danger of becoming infected with additional doses and strains of HIV as well as other sexually transmitted diseases. People who are infected with HIV and continue to use drugs or abuse alcohol or have untreated sexually transmitted diseases progress more quickly to AIDS than those who don't.

The techniques woven throughout the twelve steps can help you deal better with some of your cofactors, relax and cope with uncertainty and fear, deal more effectively with pain, sadness, and anger, become more aware of your own personal values, and find purpose and meaning in your life.

How to Use this Program

There are certain things you can do and certain things you should avoid to help keep your immune system strong and the infection in remission. These are important aspects of this program. However, it is not designed to replace your medical management program, but is to be used along with whatever other immune modulators or antiviral and antibiotic treatments you and your health care provider choose.

This book is designed to serve as an information source and a behavioral, emotional, and spiritual support. The first twelve chapters are based on the twelve steps of AA. In addition to the traditional steps they offer active coping skills, processing exercises, affirmations, relaxation, and imagery to enable you to better handle the challenges of HIV infection or AIDS. No matter what risk group you identify with or how you came to be at risk or infected, you can benefit from this material.

You can use the book in a number of ways. You may wish to actually work a twelve-step program as do the many people in AA and other twelve-step groups. In working the program most people use a sponsor, someone who is also working a twelve-step program. This person serves as a confidant and mentor. In addition to reading the book and doing the exercises, attending twelve-step meetings is helpful. If adhering to safe sex is a problem, the twelve-step meetings of Sex Addicts Anonymous or Love and Sex Addicts Anonymous may be useful. Or you may prefer to use the steps and philosophy as general guides and focus primarily on the techniques and processes. Consider this program a buffet of potentially healing tools, and, in the spirit of AA, take what you want and leave the rest. There is no right or wrong way to use this book.

If this program is your first introduction to the twelve steps you may at first find the wording of the steps, written more than fifty years ago, a bit stiff and archaic. We left the original phraseology primarily because of its clarity and directness, and because additional materials and support groups share this language. But keep in mind that you may need to stretch your literal interpretation of certain words or phrases.

Briefly, step one helps you accept where you are today. Steps two and three help you heal your relationship with a God of your understanding, a Higher Power, and develop your own spirituality. Steps four through seven help you repair your relationship with yourself; steps eight and nine help you repair your relationships with others. Steps ten, eleven and twelve serve to help maintain long-term peace of mind. The act of working the steps is never finished—there is no graduation—but rather they serve as a guide to help you live life on life's terms.

The steps are most easily worked in order from step one through step twelve, but the only essential sequence is step four before five, six before seven, and step eight before nine. It may, however, take months to finish the fourth step the first time, so most people partially work some of the other steps and use them as a general framework for their thinking and acting during this time. This will become clear as you read the various steps.

Social Support

Studies have consistently shown that, everything else being equal, people from a wide range of populations who have social support experience less morbidity (sickness) and less mortality (death) in a given time period. Studies have also shown that HIV-positive people who participate in peer groups have fewer hospital visits or incidents of high-risk behavior, and less depression. They also develop a better self-image, which promotes all aspects of health. A group can be an environment where members learn constructive coping strategies from each other, reduce isolation, and be a source of positive role models for people dealing with the same issues.

Whether you are specifically working the twelve steps or just exploring the twelve-step philosophy, you may find attending twelve-step meetings very useful and supportive. You can call your local AIDS resource center, Alcoholics Anonymous, Narcotics Anonymous, substance abuse clinics, gay, or hemophiliac organizations and ask if there are twelve-step meetings in your area for people at risk of developing HIV infection or with HIV infection. If not, you may find open AA meetings very helpful.

Keep in mind how important it is that you receive support. You may get the support you need from friends, family, a religious organization, a sponsor, a counselor, or a support group. And, although we strongly recommend the support of a group or counselor in working this program, you can work it on your own or with a friend.

Imagery, Relaxation, and Affirmations

To enhance the effectiveness of the twelve steps we have included the ancient techniques of imagery, deep relaxation, and affirmations. All three are now used extensively by many health professionals.

Imagery, the calling up of mental images designed to alter feelings and the functioning of the body, has long been employed in prayer and hypnosis, and by psychologists and shamans in many cultures. It is one of the most important ways the brain communicates with the rest of the body. Recently, the use of the relaxation response combined with imagery has become standard procedure in dealing with stress-related and chronic diseases and has proven helpful in eliminating maladaptive habits and changing physiological functioning (as in biofeedback). Athletes, executives, actors, and others use relaxation and imagery to achieve optimal performance.

The techniques of relaxation and imagery you will learn will give you an opportunity to select those images that support the mental, emotional and physical health you desire. The affirmations will help verbally and audibly reinforce new ways of feeling, thinking, and responding that enhance your well-being.

Using Imagery Scripts and Cassettes

We find the easiest and most effective way to use imagery is just to relax and listen to a tape recording of a script. For that reason we have included full scripts for each imagery in the appendix. You can make—or have someone make for you—a tape by slowly reading the script into the tape recorder with soft music playing in the background. If you choose not to use a tape, a condensed version of the script appears in this general text to help guide you.

Also for your convenience we have created a set of audiocassettes, "Living in Hope," professionally recorded using soothing background music and featuring coauthor Emmett Miller's voice. For further information, or to order, see the end of the book.

13

A Final Word

The material in this book, though well supported by scientific data, comes from our personal experiences with ourselves, our patients, and our friends. We hope what we have learned can be helpful to you. A wealth of wisdom and experience lies between these covers. Please accept it along with our love.

ONE

Awareness

STEP ONE

ADMITTED that we are **POWERLESS** over being at
risk of developing or **INFECTED** with the **AIDS VIRUS**,
that our lives have become **UNMANAGEABLE**

ADMITTED *acknowledged as true*

POWERLESS *without force or energy; devoid
of strength*

INFECTED *having had the AIDS virus enter into
the cells of one's body*

AIDS *Acquired Immune Deficiency Syndrome*

AIDS VIRUS *HIV, Human Immunodeficiency
Virus, believed to be responsible for the
suppression of the immune system, which
allows other infections, cancers, ARC (AIDS-
Related Condition), and, in its worst
expression, AIDS, to develop*

UNMANAGEABLE *without control or direction*

The first step in any twelve-step program is acceptance of your
true circumstances, no matter how devastating the circumstances may seem. This is not an attempt to consign you to despair.
Rather, acceptance of where you are is the only point from which
you can start to move forward.

Step one can help you in two ways. First, it helps you face the truth about your infection or your risk for infection. This is crucial to your health and the health of the people close to you. Second, it helps you find a deeper power that dwells within that truth. Paradoxically, through accepting your powerlessness over your infection or risk of infection and the intense feelings that accompany it, you are empowered to make changes. And once you recognize that HIV infection has made your life unmanageable, you are free to make decisions that can maximize your physical and emotional health.

Acknowledging your true circumstances is a difficult task that may bring with it rage and anguish. Yet the wisdom inherent in this step will help lighten your burden and offer you productive outlets for these feelings. (We encourage and support you for your work and struggle for having gotten this far and for being willing to enhance your well-being.)

PHIL'S STORY

Lisa had been ill since her birth. Her parents, Phil and April, had taken her to doctor after doctor, clinic after clinic. Finally the diagnosis was made. Lisa, age eighteen months, had AIDS! Phil and April were tested, and although neither of them felt sick or had any symptoms, they too were infected with HIV.

Phil had known that his hemophilia put him at risk for becoming infected by HIV-contaminated blood. But because he had had only two transfusions in his life, and had never received the concentrate (pooled serum from multiple donors containing factors deficient in hemophiliacs), he had never bothered to be tested. Although intellectually he had known he was at risk, Phil had brushed off any suspicions he had about being infected, and continued his life as usual. (This is called denial.) He had never even considered using safe sex to protect his wife, because his denial kept him from dealing with anything related to AIDS or HIV infection.

When Lisa was diagnosed with AIDS, Phil was stunned. His despair deepened when he realized he had transmitted the virus to his wife, who, in turn, had transmitted it to Lisa during the pregnancy and birth. His grief and sense of guilt at times still overwhelm him. The denial that so cunningly crept into his thinking has now severely damaged the ones he loves the most.

What Is AIDS Anyway?

AIDS stands for Acquired Immune Deficiency Syndrome. If you are HIV positive, it means your body recognized the HIV in your blood and produced antibodies against it. If you have these antibodies in your blood, your blood test will be antibody positive. If you have an antibody-positive blood test, it does *not* mean you have AIDS. It only shows that you have been infected with HIV and your body has made antibodies against HIV. Once infected, however, you have the *potential* to develop AIDS.

In reality, it is not HIV that actually causes the problems characteristic of AIDS. Considered alone, HIV is a relatively harmless virus. It is easily killed on surfaces with a dilution of one part bleach to ten parts water, and is not transmitted by casual contact. The initial infection caused by HIV is sometimes so mild people don't even notice when they become infected.

The problem is that HIV attacks your immune system, your normal defense against infection. Because the cells of your immune system can actually be killed by the virus, it can lose its ability to protect you. Viruses, fungi, and bacteria can then grow unchallenged. Such infections are called opportunistic infections because they develop only when a weakened immune system gives them the opportunity to do so. Similarly, cancers that are usually held in check may develop.

Further, if your immune system is damaged, viruses, such as the ones that caused chicken pox or cold sores when you were a child, can become reactivated. When the immune system fails, these formerly latent viruses can cause conditions such as shingles or various forms of herpes. When these opportunistic infections, cancers, or reactivated viruses, coupled with general signs and symptoms of infection, such as fevers, night sweats, and fatigue, appear, the resulting syndrome is called AIDS.

If you are already infected, your immune system needs your help. You can do many things to minimize any further weakening of your immune system and the development of certain infections.

You may be able to avoid developing AIDS. If you are not infected, your immune system needs your help to stay free of infection. Whatever your situation, this program can be useful.

Who Stays Healthy?

Most people infected with HIV are healthy. Having HIV infection does not mean you are shortly going to develop AIDS. In this first chapter we include statistics and many references to help you get a clear picture of the facts. The Centers for Disease Control (CDC) has studied men who have been infected with HIV since 1977.[1, 2] More than 45 percent are free of AIDS eleven years after infection! More than half of those who do not have AIDS or ARC have good immune lab values (T4 cell counts greater than 500). And although more than 50 percent of the seven thousand people with hemophilia in the United States became infected through transfusions before 1983, the majority of them are well.[3, 4] Despite all that we know, many aspects of the immune system remain a mystery. For example, of the children infected from transfusions as newborns, 44 percent are totally well seven years later, although 33 percent of them have severely compromised immune systems.[5] Many smaller studies show varying rates, but the major trend is consistent.

Given these statistics, you can see how accepting the truth of your situation does not mean giving in to despair; it is the first step toward learning how to stay as healthy as possible. Even if you have AIDS you can maximize your well-being by looking at the facts, gently accepting them, and then living in a health-promoting fashion.

And people who have gone on to develop AIDS differ greatly in how their bodies respond to the disease. In describing the long-term survivors (LTS), people who have actually had full-blown AIDS for longer than four years, the CDC states "only 14% of these LTS with Kaposi's sarcoma (KS) had other opportunistic diseases despite depressed immunity."[6] There are even cases where people who have tested positive for the virus have lost their antibodies to HIV and remained disease free.[7, 8]

Progression of illness varies widely depending on many things, including age, gender, risk group, geographic location, and ethnic group. Over time a general trend has been observed: women, older people, minorities, and IV drug users have shorter survival times.[9-18]

The only major change in the picture in the past few years is the increase in infection in adolescents, heterosexuals, and intravenous (IV) drug users.[19-22] It is through the IV drug users that HIV infection is gaining access to the heterosexual community and increasing in minority communities.[23-27] AIDS advances fastest in those who continue IV drug use, abuse alcohol, and/or engage in high-risk sexual behavior.[28-32] Recently an alarming increase in infection is being seen in those between the ages of thirteen and twenty-four in both the gay and the IV drug-using community. These young people felt that they were not at risk, continued high-risk behaviors, and are now showing staggering infection rates. Knowing facts such as these can help you make truly informed choices.

All in all, the statistics certainly demonstrate that becoming infected with the virus, in and of itself, is not an immediate death sentence. It is how you and your body respond to that infection that matters. You can do many things to assist your immune system. As George M. puts it, "It's similar to keeping a wound clean and dry, which hastens healing, versus picking at it, which interferes with healing." By acting in ways that can strengthen your body, rather than harm it, you give your body a chance to heal and protect itself from further damage. And the longer you live, the more likely it is you will be able to take advantage of new treatments being developed daily.

Cofactors: The Hidden Gremlins

Who becomes infected with HIV? And of those infected, who develops HIV-related illnesses? HIV can remain dormant for many years, causing no symptoms. Why do some people develop illness sooner than others or become sicker? The difference seems to involve certain cofactors.

Cofactors are conditions that occur along with the exposure to HIV or are present during HIV infection. Cofactors are also seen in many other types of illnesses. For example, smoking is a cofactor of lung cancer and anxiety is a cofactor of ulcers. Yet not everyone who smokes develops lung cancer, nor does everyone who is anxious get ulcers.

Cofactors can influence whether you become infected when exposed to HIV, as well as affect the outcome of the infection (if you get sick, when you get sick, and how sick you get).[23-42] In some way these cofactors may make getting infected easier, and if you are already infected, they may trigger the virus to become activated, thus leading to immune system supression and the development of infections or cancers. Some *suspected* cofactors include:

1. The dose of the virus (how much)

2. The strain and variant of the virus (what kind)

3. Method of transmission

4. Strength of the immune system

5. Overall physical condition, including conditions such as amoebic infections, mycoplasmas, and having had multiple treatments with antibiotics

6. Coexisting viral infections, such as hepatitis, cytomegalovirus (CMV), and various strains of herpes and chicken pox (shingles)

7. Presence of sexually transmitted diseases or genital sores or warts, especially syphilis, genital herpes, gonorrhea, or chancroid

8. Use of alcohol or mind-altering drugs

9. Length of infection at time of diagnosis and treatment

10. Gender, age, and ethnic background (may be related to socio-economic factors and access to treatment)

Controlling Your Cofactors

Some cofactors you cannot control; *others you can.* For instance, you can't alter the dose, strain, or variant of the virus you've already received, but you *do* have control over whether you get additional doses, strains, or variants. If you have any sexually transmitted diseases or other infections, you can seek treatment and protect yourself from further exposure. These are some of the ways step one can help you change: once you admit your reality, you can better direct your actions and choices.

Race and gender are other risk factors over which you obviously have no control. But armed with information and skills, you can still improve your chances. If you are a person of color, you are at increased risk for HIV infection. According to the Centers for Disease Control, around 26 percent of people with AIDS are heterosexuals. But 72 percent of these individuals are people of color.[43] Black and Hispanic adults and children are five to fifteen times more likely to become infected with HIV and become ill with AIDS than white adults and children![44,45] Studies also indicate that people of color are having a harder time eliminating their unsafe sexual practices, with syphilis on the increase, as well as the use of IV drugs.[46, 47] Lack of education and money, a feeling of hopelessness, and easy access to illegal drugs contribute to this increase.

It also seems that people of color have especially strong taboos against acknowledging that some men have sex with men. Some bisexual men of color are very ashamed and identify themselves as heterosexual, but continue having sex with unknowing women as well as men, thus spreading HIV infection to both genders.[48] Black women are forty times more likely than white women to get AIDS from an IV drug user, and four times more likely to become infected from a bisexual man. Additionally, women, especially young women of color, are becoming addicted to crack at an alarming rate, which places them at an even higher risk of developing HIV. Until recently most women became infected from having unprotected sex with infected IV drug users and bisexual men. As of 1990, more women have become infected from IV drug use than from having sex with infected men.[49-51] In 1989 AIDS was the *leading cause of death* in women aged twenty-five to thirty-four years in New York City![52]

As harsh as they are, it's important for you to accept those facts that apply to you. This awareness can prepare you to take the positive steps available. Some women, like Lisa's mother, April, did not know they were infected until they became pregnant, or until their babies were born infected. If you are HIV positive, your baby has a 30 to 50 percent chance of becoming infected, and, even if not infected, has increased chances for neonatal complications.[53, 54] Studies vary in their findings as to whether pregnancy aggravates HIV infection. But we do know that pregnancy suppresses the immune system.[55] Dormant viruses, such as genital herpes, can become reactivated at the time of delivery thus requiring that the mother have a cesarean section to protect the newborn from herpes as it passes through the infected birth canal. It is important, therefore, for women at high risk of HIV infection to know their HIV status, so they can make difficult, but at least informed, decisions regarding pregnancy.

We now know that HIV infection can be a manageable, chronic infection *if* you obtain proper diagnosis and medical management *early*. Recent findings show that the earlier the diagnosis, the better the outcome. Today there are treatments which can help prevent disease progression.[56-62]

So you can buy time, so to speak, by eliminating detrimental cofactors and by strengthening your immune system. Anything that depresses your immune system makes it easier for the disease to progress. If you do everything in your power to stay healthy, you can then benefit from new treatments. For example, Pneumocystis carinii pneumonia (PCP) a very serious pneumonia, can often be prevented by the use of inhaled medication. Until recently, PCP was the leading cause of death in people infected with HIV.

Some changes in your way of life may be required. You may need to change your diet, response to stressful situations, rest and work patterns, sleep patterns, drug or alcohol use, and sexual practices that put you at further risk. If you have not been infected, it's important to accept that certain activities place you in a position to become infected. Only you can then make a decision to avoid these activities. Unsafe sexual practices not only put *you* at risk, but also endanger the health and life of your spouse or lover. Step two further explores risky behaviors. You can imagine how badly Phil, discussed at the beginning of the chapter, must feel about infecting his wife and consequently his daughter.

It would seem logical that a person would do anything and everything to prevent disease or premature death to himself or herself or to loved ones. But this is not always the case, because the person may be in *denial*.

Denial

Denial is the act of *unconsciously* pretending to yourself or others that what is true is not true. Denial is a psychological defense mechanism that we all use to avoid pain. It can help us cope with difficult conditions we are unable to change, such as chronic pain, childhood abuse, or overwhelming loss. It is one of our most basic and valuable defense mechanisms.

But there are also dangers in denial. One danger is that when you are in denial you usually don't know it. If you find yourself avoiding certain subjects or becoming angry when those topics come up in conversation or in the media, you are probably in denial. Remember, when you're in denial, you are *unconsciously* avoiding the truth. Thus everything and everyone who represents the truth or who tries to break through your denial with the truth will probably irritate and may even enrage you. You may find parts of this book irritating when they come close to something about which you are in denial. You can use that feeling as a clue to look deeper.

The problem is denial of HIV infection or risk only works against you and others, just as it worked against Phil and his family. It can result in further damage by preventing you from changing behaviors and attitudes that are harmful. Denial of HIV infection or vulnerability to infection is just as dangerous as denial of a cancerous lump. When you are in denial, no treatment or intervention can occur; valuable time is wasted.[63, 64]

Many people respond to potentially fatal diseases with what is sometimes referred to as denial or a fighting spirit. But this type of denial—a refusal to dwell on the worst outcome—is adaptive. Denial as it refers to refusing to become consumed with negative thinking and worrying about death is useful. It is found in many long-term survivors of cancer and AIDS. It is acceptance (not denial) of the diagnosis or risk, along with a *refusal* to perceive (denial of) the condition as fatal. This kind of denial, or fighting spirit, can energize you to take the best care of yourself.

In the section to come, you will have the opportunity to discover important truths, to develop healing attitudes and healing behaviors that can prolong health and perhaps life. Occasionally, however, you may find yourself thinking, "They must be talking about somebody else; this part doesn't apply to me." This is a really dangerous trap. Please be careful and stay aware. This may be the destructive type of denial speaking!

Confronting the Crisis

The word *crisis* in Chinese is composed of two words, wu and ji. These two words mean danger and opportunity. In a crisis the wise person confronts the danger. Those who use destructive denial are running from the danger, and are incapable of seizing the opportunity. Many people have found there is opportunity in the HIV crisis. Rob is one such person.

ROB'S STORY

Rob had been an IV drug user and alcoholic for several years. He is now in recovery after going through a treatment center and a recovery home. He continues to go to AA and Narcotics Anonymous (NA) meetings, where he has many friends. Because of his high-risk behaviors, Rob knew that his chances of being infected with HIV were pretty good, but he was afraid to be tested. He knew he had shared needles with others and had been promiscuous during his using days. He couldn't imagine what he would do if he knew he was infected with the virus.

But after many long, tearful, and angry discussions with his sponsor, Rob decided to be tested. The test results were positive; he was infected. Rob's first response was one of shock and denial. He screamed at the nurse who gave him the results. "The damn lab mixed the blood up. What can you expect from a county health department!" He finally calmed down and bargained to have his blood redrawn by his private physician. The results again returned positive.

Rob was, in fact, powerless. It didn't matter how many blood tests he had or how loudly he screamed. He was infected with HIV. This time Rob was shocked out of his denial and into a rage that scared him. He ran around like a maniac, slamming doors and swearing. Rob decided that "I'm going to die soon anyway, so what the hell's the use of staying clean!"

In his rage Rob tore his apartment apart looking for any kind of drug or drink that would make him feel better. He threw his books and records at the wall. Finally, exhausted, he lay on his bed, crying. The phone rang. It was his sponsor. He came over and held Rob and gently rocked him as Rob sobbed and screamed and swore at God.

Rob came to understand that once more his life had become unmanageable, this time not because of alcohol or drugs, but because of the HIV infection and his emotional response to it. He slowly and gently allowed himself to surrender to the truth, and once again became willing to let himself be supported by others and his Higher Power. Rob decided to live just "one day at a time," as he had learned long before in AA and NA. He protected his partners by using safe sex, but disclosed his antibody test results to only a few people. His partners were impressed by his caution and pleased to find a "responsible guy for a change." He has since developed a serious relationship with Jan. He was terrified to talk to her about his infection, but felt it would be dishonest not to do so. Jan was understandably upset when Rob told her, but she remains supportive. They are still together in a deeply committed relationship.

Rob was familiar with denial; it was part of his addiction process. He had learned how to break through denial and had sought treatment for his drug and alcohol problem. This made it easier for him to come out of denial about being infected with HIV.

Denial is a natural defense against fear and pain. You gain, though, by letting it go. In denial's place you can adopt three qualities that promote your spirit and health:

- HONESTY

- OPEN-MINDEDNESS

- WILLINGNESS

These attitudes will keep you out of denial. They are frequently referred to in twelve-step programs as the HOW of the program. From time to time we will remind you of them. When we do, pause for a moment and check to see if you are continuing to maintain these qualities.

Willing to Face the Truth

Acceptance truly is the key to action and serenity. Once you accept where you are, you can move on. Denying or minimizing your reality, on the other hand, will not change it any more than an ostrich can change reality by putting its head in the sand.

If you are already infected with the virus, accepting that you are infected is incredibly tough. It can bring up enormously strong feelings of fear, loss, anger, and grief. You did not consciously choose to manage your life in such a way that you became infected with HIV, just as an alcoholic does not consciously choose to manage his life in such a way that he becomes addicted to alcohol. But the alcoholic who finally takes the first step and admits powerlessness over alcohol then has the freedom to surrender and not drink, one day at a time.

It may sound strange at first, but the relief that comes with that acceptance is quite remarkable. For the alcoholic there is no more trying to drink like a normal person, and there is a newfound energy that comes from giving up that attempt. It is the surrender into powerlessness that is behind the AA saying that you can choose to run the disease rather than have the disease run you.

Similarly, once you are able to accept that you are infected and the feelings that come with that knowledge, then all the energy previously spent on denial and fighting will become available to you. Although you are powerless over the virus, you are not powerless over how your body and your mind respond to the virus. Likewise, you are powerless over the intense feelings, but you are not powerless over how you deal with them. Like the alcoholic, you can choose to run the disease—to find healthy, satisfying responses—rather than allowing the disease to run you—limiting yourself unnecessarily in spirit, mind, and body. Now you have choices, and it is these choices around which this program is designed. As you discovered in the Introduction, there are concrete actions you can take that can help strengthen your physical and emotional responses. There are also ways you can protect yourself from further damage. You may not be able to control the disease totally, but you can certainly do many things to affect its course.

If you are not infected but are in a group that is at high risk for becoming infected, accepting that can be just as difficult as

26

accepting HIV infection. It is, however, just as important. You are powerless over the virus. You cannot control how the virus infects people or whom it infects. But once you accept you are at high risk for infection, you have the power to choose to engage in behaviors that prevent infection. You can choose to minimize your risk of becoming infected. You too are powerless over your emotions, but you can choose responses that use these intense emotions for your benefit, rather than your harm.

HIV infection is not a highly contagious infection. It is, simply put, a behavioral infection. If you do not engage in the behaviors that transmit the virus, you will not become infected. Until recently, not all behaviors and transmission routes were known, so many people did not have the choices that we have today.

Antibody Testing

Another choice that you have today is finding out whether you are infected with HIV. It is an excellent way to break through denial. We know a number of people in high-risk groups who were nervous wrecks until they had the HIV antibody test. Some were very relieved to find out they were not infected. They then changed their behavior to make sure that they did not become infected. By accepting the dangers, they created an opportunity to preserve their health. They actively dealt with their feelings and are no longer constantly anxious.

Others found out that they were infected. They experienced shock, anger, grief, fear, and the other feelings that are evoked by such a discovery. Before being tested, however, many had been almost certain their tests would come out positive.[65] Until they were certain, though, they avoided making any changes, because to do so would mean confronting that terrible reality. After confirming their suspicions, they told us that the not knowing had been harder and had caused more distress than the knowing. [66–68] They then made real commitments and dedicated efforts to change their behavior and deal with their feelings in healthy ways.[69, 70]

Most of them are now daily dealing with life on life's terms. They are working through their emotions and striving for an accepting and energetic attitude. They avoid activities that could make them sick, and try to engage only in those that promote health. They now feel more in charge of their lives. Some have even told us that becoming infected with HIV was a blessing in disguise, because it acted as a positive force in their lives. A door was opened to new ways of feeling, new ways of appreciating and interacting with themselves and others.

If you are in a high-risk group and have either not had the test done or have not returned for your results, we urge you to do so. The National Hemophiliac Foundation is recommending that all people who received blood products *and* their sexual partners be tested, and, if positive, have their immune systems monitored every three to six months. It also makes some suggestions for treatment alternatives. The Foundation representatives feel so strongly that they state, "If you choose not to be tested, you and your physician should *assume* that you are infected with HIV."[71]

It is essential that you know exactly where you stand, and it is important to find out as soon as possible. The earlier the treatment, the better the outcome, and the longer a person is infected with the virus, the *more contagious* he or she bcomes. Some sexual partners of hemophiliacs who had not been infected with the virus in 1983 are today testing positive. Lulled into complacency and denial by their previous negative test results, they failed to adopt low-risk behaviors and then became infected. Those who adopted safe sex practices have prevented transmission to their partners.[72]

Once you get your results you can stop worrying and find out what you need to do to best help yourself and loved ones. Information and counseling are available before and after you get the test results. We strongly encourage you to take advantage of both. It is best to write down your questions before going to be sure you remember them and can have them all answered. The information can be very valuable in increasing your understanding of your options and allaying your fears. Counseling will also allow you to express your feelings.

If you're unsure of how you'll react to your test results, don't dwell on the thought of it. Just take this process one step at a time. You will be able to handle the information, and you will eventually be glad you found out. The information in this book can really help you deal with whatever occurs. People who find they are infected with the virus often abandon high-risk behaviors.[73, 74]

Chances are excellent that your life can improve in many ways you can't even imagine right now.

If you are in a treatment facility for drug or alcohol abuse, we suggest you discuss your concerns regarding HIV infection with your counselor. For many people, dealing with substance abuse is difficult enough. Adding the strain of antibody testing may be too much, too soon. You may do better getting tested later, after you have developed a strong support system in the recovering community. You may, however, live in an area where infection rates are high or be so worried about your HIV status that getting tested while in a treatment or a recovery facility is to your advantage. There you are in a structured environment and supported by professionals to help you work through the feelings that arise. In this way you can come to accept and surrender to two big chunks of truth, your addiction and possible HIV infection, where trained personnel can assist you in developing strategies for a new and safer life after discharge.

Each person is different however, and only you and your counselors know what's best for you at any particular point in time. Many treatment programs are offering testing and find that it is very helpful and the worry that it would cause people to relapse into drug or alcohol abuse is not the case—they actually were better able to avoid drug/alcohol abuse.[75-80]

Regardless of whether you decide to be tested or not; are positive or negative—remember the way you *get* and the way you *give* HIV and other infections is by those high-risk activities described in step two.

If you test negative for the HIV antibody, guard against denying your risks. High-risk behaviors are still high-risk behaviors. It is true that some people become infected after only one exposure, while others don't after many exposures. We don't have all the answers but suspect the cofactors previously listed have a lot to do with this fact. There is no known natural immunity to HIV and people who were not infected before but continued high-risk behaviors became infected later. Playing Russian roulette with your life just isn't worth it. There are people who will support your new decisions and way of life and celebrate your changing to safer activities. Sticking with them will make your commitment much easier.

Are you in a high-risk group? You are if you are:

1. a man who has sex with other men

2. an IV drug user

3. a hemophiliac

4. a blood transfusion recipient between 1979 and March 1985

5. a sexual partner of any of the above

6. a sexual partner of a person with many sexual partners

If you test positive to the HIV antibody:

1. You have been exposed to and infected with HIV, and your body has created antibodies to fight it.

2. You are contagious and can pass the virus to others during sex or by sharing needles.

3. *It does not necessarily mean you are sick now or will definitely get sick or get AIDS in the near future.*

If you test negative to the HIV antibody, it means one of the following:

1. You have not been exposed to the virus.

2. You have been exposed to the virus, but have not become infected.

3. You have been infected, but your body has not yet produced antibodies to the HIV. Most people who are infected will develop a positive test within six weeks, but if you are in a high-risk group and test negative, it is recommended that you be retested in two months and again in six months.

Alcohol and Drugs: More Cofactors

The use of alcohol and drugs influences the state of your health. A recent report from Hahnemann University in Philadelphia says that even "moderate drinking may speed the development of full-fledged AIDS in people who have been infected but show no symptoms of the disease." Accepting this fact is part of the first step. It may seem drastic or difficult, but ignoring the facts doesn't make them go away. Please call on your honesty, open-mindedness, and willingness to help you through any reluctance to believe this.

We have known for some time that the use of alcohol can have a direct negative effect on the immune system, resulting in increased infections and increased death from these infections.[81] Alcohol suppresses immune function long before it causes any liver damage or nutritional deficiencies. It has a profound effect on the spleen and thymus[82] and interferes with antibody production and the number and function of white blood cells (WBCs).[80] Therefore, if your immune system is already under attack, drinking even moderate amounts of alcohol makes no sense. Alcohol also negates the effects of antibiotics. Drinkers whose infections clear up while they are in the hospital find their infections return after they go home and resume drinking. Antibiotics can't work as they were intended if alcohol is in your body.

The effects of other recreational drugs on the immune system have been documented more recently. For example, even in extremely small doses, THC, the psychoactive chemical in marijuana, inhibits the cells of your immune system in their most fundamental activities. (The macrophage, an important WBC, is impaired in its ability to move and digest bacteria and in its ability to produce interleukin 1, a vital component of the immune system's arsenal against retroviruses, including HIV.[83] THC suppresses the activity of other WBCs, which are instrumental in fighting off cancers, and interferes with the production of antibodies, interleukins, and interferons.) All of the cells of your immune system, and the substances they secrete, are vital to your remaining free of infection and disease. If you continue to smoke marijuana you are specifically destroying the very cells and substances you need to stay healthy while putting your mind at risk of extra disturbance.[84-87]

Using amphetamines (speed) is especially harmful to your immune system. Cocaine has actually been shown to activate the virus, and the use of crack and cocaine is the biggest predictor of which IV drug users become infected.[88-94] Various forms of speed, including "poppers" (amyl nitrate), used to be the recreational drug of choice in the gay community.[74, 95, 96] The prognosis for people who continue to use speed, especially crack or cocaine, is the worst of all. Speed exhausts your body and keeps stress chemicals racing around inside it, and while "speeding" you can forget to eat and sleep properly and may be inclined to go on a "speed and sex run."

Anything that alters your mind and your perceptions will make it harder for you to change old behaviors. As an example, in the gay male population, heavy drinkers are twice as likely to become infected as moderate drinkers or nondrinkers, and the use of drugs and alcohol remains the strongest predictor of infection in young gay men and of relapse to unsafe sex.[97-103]

Also, it is important to remember there is a cross-addiction between drugs and alcohol. This leads many people who have stopped drinking to become addicted to drugs. Likewise, many addicts who have stopped using drugs but continue to drink alcohol find they abuse alcohol, and that when drunk they start using drugs again. It is the same disease wrapped in a different package. Alcohol is just a drug in liquid form that today happens to be legal!

The abuse of steroids is a drug problem sometimes seen in the gay community. The emphasis on physical appearance and the obsession with body-building has led some gay men to use steroids to "bulk up." Steroids are very suppressive of the immune system! If you are on steroids without a good medical reason we suggest you get to a doctor fast to taper off them. You cannot just stop. If you have been on steroids for any length of time, you need to gradually reduce your intake or you could have a fatal shutdown of your adrenal glands!

For those of you who are at risk of becoming infected or became infected with the virus through IV drugs, stopping your drug use can help you keep an HIV infection from shortly progressing to full-blown AIDS. Even people on a methadone maintenance program do much better than people who continue injecting drugs.[104-106]

You do have a choice. As an IV drug user, your immune system is already damaged by the drugs you use.[107-110] Your white blood cells recognize "nonself" particles, such as viruses, bacteria, and drugs, and then try to destroy them. When you use drugs your white blood cells are too busy trying to figure out what it is you just injected into your bloodstream to effectively do their job.

People who are HIV positive and continue to shoot drugs have very poor outcomes. But many people have kicked their addiction with help. Many people have used a twelve-step program to do that; others have avoided HIV infection and AIDS through methadone maintenance programs.[111, 112] Some have done both. There are some Narcotics Anonymous (NA) meetings now specifically for people on methadone.

We realize that there is a shortage of treatment centers, especially in major cities. If you cannot get into a treatment center right away, do yourself a favor and get on a waiting list as soon as possible. While you are waiting, please *don't share needles* with anyone, not even your sexual partner! If you find that impossible, clean your "works" with plain old household bleach before and after sharing. It takes only a minute. Just draw up bleach through the needle, fill the syringe, and squirt it out. Do this twice. Then rinse the syringe and needle the same way twice with water. And don't share your water; it can be contaminated with blood. While you are waiting to get into treatment, NA meetings can be very helpful.

If you do not abuse drugs or alcohol, it is still wise to refrain from their use. Everyone we talked with said how important it was for them to avoid alcohol abuse and drug use. A few people, who have never had a problem with drugs or alcohol, continue to have a drink on special occasions. In trying for balance in their lives they avoid being too rigid in any area. People with no history of abuse still have this option. If, however, you have abused alcohol or drugs, even a glass of wine or one small joint may set off a compulsion and lead to abuse.

Any amount probably harms your immune system. One study shows the consumption of approximately three cans of beer causes increased replication of the HIV for at least one and one-half days.[113] Others show how alcohol advances the progression of disease in infected individuals.[32, 114] If you find that you are having a hard time stopping, or find yourself making excuses for why you continue to drink or use drugs, please closely examine your use and consider that you might be addicted. Denial can be deadly.

You don't need to be arrested for drunk driving, be fired from your job, or go to jail to have a problem with drugs or alcohol. The old stereotype of the down-and-out person on Skid Row is by no means the most common type of alcoholic or addict. Most are teaching in schools, working in hospitals, playing professional sports, or running corporations. Like being infected with HIV, addiction is a disease. No one chooses to get it. But you can't do anything about a problem until you admit you've got it.

If you are homosexual or bisexual, you are especially at risk for alcoholism or drug addiction. In the general population, one out of seven people are alcoholics or addicts, but in the homosexual community studies consistently indicate one out of three are alcoholics or addicts.[115-119] The professionals who treat HIV-infected people are usually aware that these people frequently have a personal history of drug or alcohol abuse and frequently have a family history of alcohol abuse.[114, 120] The gay community *used* to support that kind of behavior and socialization.

The following questions are compiled from several different lists used to help a person determine whether he or she is an alcoholic or drug addict. If you answer yes to any two of these questions, chances are good that you are an alcoholic or a drug addict. If you answer yes to three or more, you are most likely an alcoholic or a drug addict and need total abstinence.

SELF-TEST

1. Do you lose time from work or school as a result of your drinking or using drugs?

2. Is drinking or using drugs making your home life unhappy?

3. Do you drink or use drugs to overcome shyness or to feel more at ease with other people?

4. Have you gotten into financial difficulties as a result of drinking or using drugs?

5. Has anyone—family, friends, co-workers, doctor, or mental health care provider—suggested that you have a problem with drinking or using drugs?

6. Does your drinking or using drugs make you careless or forgetful of the welfare of yourself, your family, or your friends?

7. Do you find yourself wanting a drink or drug at a definite time of the day or the "morning after"?

8. Do you drink or use drugs to escape from worries or troubles?

9. Do you drink or use drugs alone?

10. Have you ever had a complete loss of memory while drinking or using drugs?

11. Do you find that you do things when you are drinking or using drugs that you wouldn't otherwise do and of which you are later ashamed?

12. Do you try to control your use of alcohol or drugs by making promises to yourself or others—only to later break them?

13. Do you engage in risky behaviors or go to dangerous places when drinking or using drugs?

You just cannot choose life and continue to get high or loaded. Your immune system can't take it. If you respond with, "What the hell, why not," that may be the denial of alcoholism or drug addiction speaking for you. It's an unconscious response. You see, chemical addiction is the only disease that tells you that you don't have a disease. Remember, the moment you put a drug or alcohol into your body, *your mind is no longer your own!* You now have a drug running your mind and telling you there is no problem.

That is why substance abuse is called the disease of denial. And that is also why it is so hard to break the denial. The exact thing that you need to do to get well—think straight—is made impossible by the drug.

If you have recognized a problem and decided to do something about it, you have probably made the best and hardest decision of your life. One recovering addict/alcoholic says, "I realized that my addiction was going to kill me long before the AIDS virus could." Please call and get a list of meetings or just to talk. You may feel exhausted after finally making the decision to get help. The sections that follow discuss positive self-talk and deep relaxation, and can help you to be more centered. Take some deep breaths and read on.

Positive Self-Talk

Positive self-talk (also called affirmations) is very important. Your deeper mind listens carefully to everything you say, out loud or in your mind. This self-talk can either help heal or help destroy your self-esteem, your self-image, and even your health. It is a self-fulfilling prophecy: if you call yourself stupid, or someone else important to you calls you stupid, long enough, you start to believe it, and start acting stupid. Soon that is all anyone, including yourself, expects, and you seem to have become stupid even though you really are not.

It is as if we each have the seeds within us to be many different types of people. It is the seed that gets nourished that grows and blooms. We nourish that seed by self-talk and reinforcement from those around us. Whatever is focused on simply becomes bigger. Though we are not aware of it, self-talk goes on constantly. It's important to become aware of your self-talk and change it to what you *want* to be true. You can change your thoughts and your reality by focusing on what messages you constantly feed your mind.

At first positive self-talk may sometimes feel awkward and dishonest. You may not feel at all like what the statement says. Try to be patient and trust that somewhere, in some way, that statement *can* be true for you. Somewhere within you lies the seed for this kind of reality. Over time you will feel more comfortable with the affirmation and understand it more deeply. Affirmations are directions in which you are headed that are stated in the present as if they are already true. They are the blueprint for new ways of being and acting; repeating them waters the seed of a healthy and lovable you.

A very effective way to use affirmations is to read them into a tape recorder and listen to and repeat them several times a day. As a reminder you can also copy them and post them in prominent places, such as on your bathroom mirror.

POSITIVE SELF-TALK

- I deserve the best.

- If I don't think I deserve the best or don't want the best for myself now, by the time I get further into this program I will feel differently.

- If I suspect I have an addiction to drugs or alcohol I can accept that possibility and call for help!

- I can be kind to myself and my body.

- Surrendering to what *is* allows me to go forward.

- I cannot control the virus, but I *can* control my behavior and my body's response to the virus.

- I accept full responsibility for myself and my here and now.

- I choose to accept the truth.

Deep Relaxation and Imagery: The Loving Light

The loving light is the most basic imagery exercise. It will help you let go of some of the physical and emotional tension that may have developed as you have been reading this chapter on the first step. Relaxation and imagery are vital aspects of this program. They will help you eliminate excessive anxiety and fear while allowing you to develop focused concentration.

Imagery is one of the most important ways the brain communicates with the body. You can't will yourself to salivate like you can will yourself to move your hand. But if you imagine squeezing some lemon juice into a glass for a few moments, and then imagine drinking the sour lemon juice, you will start producing saliva. When you focus your thoughts an image forms. It is represented in the brain by a specific pattern. This pattern then influences deeper structures in the nervous system, which in turn affect emotions, behaviors, and other normally unconscious systems, such as the immune and glandular systems (including the salivary glands).

Imagery is powerful because the brain and body will respond to an image in a manner that is consistent with the image. Salivation is consistent with lemon juice. If you hold an image of ants and fleas crawling all over your body, the response will be a feeling of itchiness. Similarly, if you hold the image of yourself as helpless and hopeless, your body will start slouching and have a tendency to just give up. If you see yourself as trapped, your body will become tight and tense owing to the chemicals secreted.

Imagery is a skill that develops with practice. Try not to judge your imagery. Everyone's is different. Some people see vivid pictures in their minds; others hear words or music or feel movements or emotions. When visualizing a loving light, you may prefer to see a white light or a golden light—or a green, orange, or purple light. Tomorrow that may change. Go with whatever happens for you.

The words we offer have no special magic. It is the images triggered in your mind that work the magic. As time goes on you will feel more comfortable working with imagery. Your images combined with positive self-talk can help you reach a truly calm and comfortable place despite external circumstances.

After some practice you will be able to repeat the steps from memory, and use them to deeply relax any time you want to calm yourself. Begin each imagery exercise found in this book with a five- to ten-minute period of deep relaxation as discussed in Part 1 of this exercise. A full script is on page 282 if you want to make a tape.

Repeat this exercise one to three times a day, especially any time you feel frightened, tense, or angry, until you reach the next imagery exercise in this book. The most effective times are first thing in the morning, midday, and right before going to sleep at night.

Before you start, eliminate any possibility of interruption or distraction so that you can focus completely upon relaxation, upon peace, and upon your own healing. Unplug the phone, put a sign on the door, let people know you are going to be taking some time for your own healing and unstressing. Empty your bladder, get a blanket and pillow, loosen any constricting clothing, and sit or lie comfortably in a quiet place. Begin by letting yourself become aware that at this moment there is no place you have to go, nothing you have to do, and no problem you have to solve. Take a few moments now to do this.

Part 1: Deep Relaxation

Breathe in as deeply as is comfortable, and with each breath out, count, starting with the number 1, and breathe twenty slow, deep breaths. This deep breathing is a signal to your brain that all is well and that it is okay to stop producing stress chemicals. For this reason it is used to begin most types of meditation techniques.

Now imagine that beneath your feet is a globe of light. The bottoms of your feet are hollow, allowing the light to flow into your feet. Imagine your entire body filling with light, peace, relaxation, and love, from the bottoms of your feet to the top of your head.

Feel the light coming out of the top of your head, surrounding you from head to toe. The outside of this cocoon of light is polished smooth like a mirror and reflects all negative energy away from you. You are within this cocoon, and its positive healing energy soothes and nurtures you.

Tell yourself that any time during the day or night, you can take a deep breath in and bring this relaxed feeling back by just imagining that the bottoms of your feet are hollow and that there is a globe of light beneath your feet. Then, as you slowly breathe in, that soft, healing light caressingly calms and heals you wherever you are.

Any time unnecessary thoughts enter your mind, simply let the light flow into that part of your mind and clear away the thoughts. Imagine that you are a being of light and that at your center you sense a Higher Power, which brings you healing, wholeness, and peace.

Part 2: Opening to the Light

Guide this healing light into the deepest parts of your being. First, feel it flowing into your mind, bringing clear thinking, accurate memory, and positive thoughts. Repeat silently several times:

- Today I make and act on decisions that nurture me.

- I am capable of acting and thinking in new ways.

- I can concentrate and focus on my intentions and follow through on them.

- Today I speak clearly and say what I truly mean to say.

And as the soft light gently washes away all doubts, all negative thinking, guide the healing light into your feelings and emotions and silently repeat:

- Today I recognize that my feelings are only feelings; I do not have to act on them.

- I can feel my feelings. They are a part of me. My feelings will not harm me.

- Deep within I feel in harmony; balance and enlightened in my spirit.

- Today I can deal with, and grow from, anger and sadness, even fear and depression.

- Today I can be with my feelings, for I have an inner and an outer source of strength.

- Today I have within me a bottomless well, a limitless source, of hope and energy.

And with each breath, let that gentle light of relaxation, love, and healing flow into every part of your body as you repeat silently:

- I open my head, face, and neck to the healing light and feel all tensions melting away.

- I open my back and chest and breathe the healing light into every cell of my body.

- I open my heart and allow the healing light to flow in, and today I feel my heart being healed.

- I open my arms and hands and feel them growing more powerful and vital.

- I open my abdomen, pelvis, and genitals to the healing light and feel its warmth working within me.

- I open my legs and feet to the healing light, and feel them growing stronger.

- With each breath my body grows more vital.

- Today I know how to relax and nurture myself, and I choose to do it often.

And now bring to mind an image of the most relaxing, comfortable, and healing place you can think of; a place far away from anything that could disturb you; a place where you can let yourself be totally at peace. It might be a place you've been, or a place you've always wanted to go, or an imaginary place.

Now imagine yourself drifting through space and time, as though you are riding on a magic carpet to this special place. And as you arrive, begin picturing the sights; see what is around you in full color. Let yourself imagine you can hear the sounds, smell the smells, and feel the temperature. Bring in all the details you can; really let yourself be there.

And as you drift into this most wonderful place, imagine your body as healthy and as well as you can picture; your muscles strong, your mind clear, your emotions balanced, and your entire being feeling very whole. How wonderful it is!

Part 3: Reawakening

Imagine that you have become the person you really want to be, with the mental, physical, emotional, and spiritual health you really want to have.

And now, slowly, over a period of about thirty seconds, let yourself gradually return to a wide awake awareness of the space around you. Come back feeling rested, energized, and healed. Or, if you wish, you can let yourself continue to rest, or even drift off into a deep, rejuvenating sleep.

Staying in the Present

The single most valuable tool to help you deal with your risk of infection with HIV and the subsequent emotions is the concept of staying in the present moment. This means keeping your awareness focused on feelings and events as they occur. If you are also addicted to drugs or alcohol, this tool is crucial to recovery, as the millions of people in twelve-step programs have come to know. Using it marks the start of managing your life energy in healthy, fulfilling ways. Here is one of the readings commonly found in twelve-step literature:

YESTERDAY—TODAY—TOMORROW

There are two days in every week about which we need not worry, two days which should be kept free from fear and apprehension. One of these days is *yesterday*, with its mistakes and cares, its faults and blunders, its aches and pains. *Yesterday* has passed forever beyond our control. All the money in the world cannot bring back *yesterday*. We cannot undo a single act we performed; we cannot erase a single word we said . . . *yesterday* is gone.

The other day we need not worry about is *tomorrow*, with its possible adversities, its burdens, its large promise and poor performance. *Tomorrow* is also beyond our immediate control. *Tomorrow's* sun will rise, either in splendor or behind a mask of clouds—but it will rise. Until it does, we have no stake in *tomorrow,* for it is as yet unborn.

This leaves only one day ... *today.* Anyone can fight the battle of just one day. It is only when you and I add the burdens of those two awful eternities—*yesterday* and *tomorrow*—that we break down. It is not the experience of *today* that drives men mad—it is remorse and bitterness for something which happened *yesterday* and the dread of what *tomorrow* may bring.

LET US, THEREFORE, LIVE BUT ONE DAY AT A TIME!

Letting go of the past and dropping worry about the future gives you more energy and vitality to spend in the present, which is the only time you can really use it. A twelve-step program helps you learn how to live one day at a time. Remember that the only time anyone is guaranteed is the now. And time is nothing more than an infinite succession of "nows."

Try bringing yourself back to the present every time you find your thoughts wandering to the past or the future. Ask yourself, "Where am I right now? What am I doing? Is it good for me?" Notice how it feels.

How do you feel about today? Can you recognize any blessings in your life right now? It may sound strange, but there really are some blessings. When you feel overwhelmed it's easy to forget them.

Stop for a moment now. How do you feel? What is your truth right this very second? Many of us aren't even aware of where we are at any point in time because our minds stay so busy somewhere else. Bringing your attention to the present lets you release the stress that may otherwise go unnoticed until it causes enough discomfort to stop you. What about that muscle that's just starting to tighten, the anxious thought that needs acknowledging and letting go? Staying in the present and turning your attention to your inner experience allows you to dump any ill effect from a stressful event as soon as it starts.

Positive Self-Talk: Staying in the Present

Employing the following affirmations is a powerful means of supporting your staying in the present. Staying in the present helps you work through the feelings that will surface when doing this difficult first step. Feelings that would have felt overwhelming can be handled when taken *one minute at a time.*

- I can choose to stay in the truth, and to tap into the power of the present moment.

- I have power over the present.

- The past is unchangeable.

- The future is beyond my grasp unless I keep my mind centered in the here and now.

- I can be calm and serene.

Stages of Acceptance

The six stages a person typically goes through when confronted with any loss or painful discovery, whether it be a positive HIV test result, a diagnosis of AIDS, or a death or divorce, are *shock, denial, bargaining, fear, anger* and *acceptance.* These stages can vary in order and intensity, and may come and go, depending on the individual. You can also be in more than one stage at the same time. You may think you've worked through all of your anger or fear, but when circumstances change, find yourself in anger or fear again. *That does not mean you are regressing or doing anything wrong.* We all recycle feelings around highly charged situations; it is the nature of the process. Sometimes your moods may swing so quickly that they scare you. One minute you may feel completely accepting and calm, and the next minute you may be overflowing with rage. Please be gentle with yourself. This happens to everyone, even the most balanced and spiritual of people.

We've already seen examples of shock and denial. The bargaining phase is the phase of, "If I say a novena, become a vegetarian, and meditate every day for two hours, maybe my test results will change." There is no real harm in this, provided it does not lead to compulsive behavior or ongoing denial.

Fear

Fear, however, can sometimes be paralyzing. The saying, "Fear is lack of faith," may be true. But it is also true that fear is part of the human experience. Some self-righteous people pride themselves on their "faith that allows no room for fear." We suspect that anyone who claims to be free of *all* fear, *all* of the time, is probably in denial or dishonest. People are frequently reluctant to admit fear because they think that they should be above it, or that it means they lack a trust in God.

Fear is a natural response, designed to protect you from danger. This is fine when fear prevents you from walking into a fire. But when fear prevents you from looking at a truth, or the avoidance of a fear-provoking situation prevents you from going through the emotional pain of growth, then fear becomes a liability.

When you find yourself in fear, please don't beat yourself up. There is nothing wrong with being afraid. That doesn't mean that fear is not painful. Fear is terribly uncomfortable: that's why many of us have tried medicating away the pain of fear. But humans have human feelings, and fear is just one of them. Avoid judging yourself and questioning your faith.

Consider Jesus. Whether you believe the Bible is an inspired work or an interesting book, whether you consider Jesus your personal Savior or a fascinating character, his example of a human under extreme stress is a good one. It is said that when he was in the garden the night before the crucifixion, he was in such fear that he cried and sweat blood. So if this figure could have such fear, who are we to think we should be above it? It may be true that the only thing to fear is fear itself, but as long as we are human we will experience fear.

The path to acceptance and emotional healing is one of allowing the fear, or, as Eastern philosophers put it, embracing the fear. In order to embrace the fear you need to first accept that you have it. Feel that knot in your gut or notice the fluttering in your chest and address it. "What have we here? Oh, it's fear. That's okay, it means I'm still alive and still human. All humans experience fear.

Today I'm going to accept my humanity and allow myself to feel this fear without feeling ashamed. If Jesus could cry bloody tears and cry out from the cross 'Why have you forsaken me?' I guess I can still love myself, stomach knots, heart palpitations, and all." The sooner you embrace your fear, the sooner it will lose its power over you.

One special kind of fear is worry. If you find yourself worrying, you are in the future. Stop and ask yourself, "Is there anything I can do about this (the thing you are worrying about) right now, right this moment?" If there is, go ahead and do it. If there isn't, tell yourself that: "There is nothing I can do about that now. Instead of worrying I choose to occupy my mind with something else."

Your mind can concentrate on only one thing at a time. So acknowledge whatever your body feels (My stomach is tense) and bring your thoughts to your immediate reality (I'm here, alive and safe at this moment. Is there anything I can do right this very moment? Yes, I can take deep breaths and relax myself.) Centering yourself emotionally, physically, and mentally in this way frees up your spirit. The loving light exercise can help you do this.

If despite all this you continue to find yourself worrying, try doing something with your mind or your body. Call or visit someone, write about or to the fear, sing, chant, go for a walk and whistle, sort through drawers, or organize your tapes and records. Move your body and change your thoughts. But *do* something!

Shame and Anger

To free up more of your energy, it helps to work through the anger and grief that inevitably surround HIV infection. If you acquired the virus through some sexual or drug-related behavior in which you willingly participated, it is useful to look at those choices and accept responsibility for them. You may not have even known the choice placed you at risk for acquiring HIV, but nonetheless, accepting responsibility for making that choice has a purpose. Response-ability is not at all the same as blame. It merely means looking at the truth and learning from it so you have the ability to choose a different response in the future.

If you knew you were placing yourself at risk, you may feel

guilt: the natural response when you see yourself not living up to your standards. Try to allow yourself to feel it. You can use the guilt to empower yourself to do things differently in the future. It is important, however, to then forgive yourself and let go of it. Staying stuck in the guilt is a seductive form of denial in which self-punishment takes the place of responsible action. This self-punishment then weakens you more and sets you up for more poor choices and less responsibility.

Keep in mind that all you did was make a poor and dangerous choice. We all have made poor choices in our lifetimes, and most of us have also made dangerous ones. We are not trying to minimize the heavy price tag that may come with such a choice. But remember, that is all it was—a poor choice—and there is no shame in that. Shame says, I am bad at my core, worthless and incapable of doing the right thing. It is also a form of denial that leads to avoidance of responsibility. If I am basically incapable and bad, I can't be expected to respond in healthy ways.

Many of us have deep feelings of shame that originated in childhood. We can slip into feeling shame easily and quickly and not even recognize it as shame. All we know is that we suddenly feel depressed or anxious.

You can learn to use the guilt and let go of the shame. Millions of people have learned to do this. The twelve steps is one way to do it. Otherwise, your shame can deceive you and stand in the way of your accepting responsibility for yourself and doing what you need to take care of yourself. Handling the guilt and shame breaks the depression and gives you back your power!

The feeling that can really be useful is the feeling of anger. When you can stop turning your anger into blame of self or others you can feel it for what it is. You may not be infected yourself, but still feel intense anger. You are powerless over the emotions that automatically come with this kind of situation. It's normal to feel these intense feelings. You are not, however, powerless over what you choose to do with these feelings. The way in which you deal with these feelings is very important.

Not every person is even aware of his or her anger. But it's a natural part of experiencing loss, and it usually burns brightest after we come out of our initial shock, denial, bargaining, and fear. Some of us give free expression to rage. Others have learned to clip the wings of anger. We cage it inside, fearing we will lose control if we let it out. It is more healthy to let our anger out, to let its vitality fill us. You can provide a safe outlet for it by creating a specific physical setting and means to aid you: a punching bag, tennis racket, plastic bat, or pillows. This may feel a bit artificial and awkward at first, but it can help immensely in releasing anger's chemicals and muscular effects.

Anger arises from the awareness of one's own intrinsic value, and leads to the reassertion of the self. It is a very powerful emotion, one intended to move you into action. Anger gives you the strength to do things that otherwise you might not do. It can carry you, phoenixlike, out of the ashes of the past and into a rich future. Denial of your anger allows it to turn inward and become depression, which can further impair your immune function. In allowing expression of your anger, you turn away from feelings of helplessness, which would cast you as victim. Many people we talked with have used their anger to energize them to work on political, emotional, or medical issues associated with AIDS. They have made a remarkable contribution, and many of the services now available would not exist were it not for these people's positive use of their anger.

The Victim Stance

Many people who are infected come out of the initial stages and go through a "Why me?" stage. That's a perfectly normal and understandable response to this devastating news. This phase usually passes quickly, but may return for short, intermittent periods. If you acquired the virus from blood or blood products, artificial insemination, donated organs, unconsenting sex, or sex with someone who did not tell you he or she was infected, you may find this stance an especially tempting one. You may even be supported in this stance by uninformed and well-intentioned friends or family.

Every person infected with HIV is a victim, and every person infected with HIV deserves sympathy and consolation. But every person infected with HIV who *stays* in the victim role is sabotaging himself or herself! You may consider yourself a victim of an awful twist of fate, and thinking and feeling like a victim can be justified and rationalized in several ways. But to regain control of your circumstances, and to create the best possible life for yourself, it is important to move on.

You are powerless over the fact that you are infected with HIV or at risk for becoming infected, just as you are powerless over the feelings that arise because of this. But you have choices about how your life proceeds from here. If you accept this, you can take one step after another to strengthen your immune system, your inner life, and your honesty, openness, and willingness relative to your truth, to yourself, and to others, starting right now. This includes recognizing your anger, being willing to experience the anger fully, and expressing the anger in ways that add to your life.

If you keep seeing yourself as a victim, you will not complete the experience of your rage, and cannot redirect it to feel truly vital, powerful, and whole. Avoid the temptation to play martyr or to try to look good! To choose to remain a victim is to choose to be helpless and hopeless.

You can decide to graduate from the victim stance and escape this potential downward spiral. Because you are reading this, you are already in the process of promoting yourself to the status of survivor. You may feel only a flicker of hope from this right now, or you may feel a "So what?" emptiness. If so, don't worry. You have already lived through a major loss. Feelings of numbness and emptiness may come and go for some time.

But if feelings of helplessness and hopelessness persist and no one or nothing has any positive effect on you for an extended period of time (weeks or months), take them seriously and please get professional help. If you lose weight owing to lack of appetite, or if you find yourself crying continuously or seriously contemplating suicide, seek help. It's important that clinical depression be managed by you and a professional, and it is common for people to experience periods of true depression because of HIV infection.

This program can help you avoid prolonged depression. It offers a process for living through your anger and grief. Another way to stay out of depression is to have support from understanding, loving people.

Support Groups

The thought of discussing your deep thoughts and feelings with a group of strangers might be uncomfortable at first, but a support group can be a great source of energy, comfort, and understanding. We strongly recommend them and especially suggest twelve-step program groups. You can get a list of local support groups from your local AIDS hotline or AIDS project.

Studies indicate that individuals who have strong social support have reduced psychological distress and enhanced recovery from serious illness.[75, 121] Papers presented at the Fourth International Conference on AIDS discuss how self-help and peer groups help alleviate isolation and counteract depression.[122, 131] In a group of HIV-infected individuals, loneliness was associated with diminished immune system activity by several different measures.[75, 132]

Just as companies hire consultants when they deal with certain issues, you can give yourself an advantage by seeking out people whose experience may offer you new insights. It is really helpful to have a place where you can go and share your feelings and thoughts; spending time with people who are in the same or a similar situation can ease your life immeasurably. Through this common bond you can assist and nurture each other.[133] This is the basis on which AA was founded.

Support groups do not, however, take the place of professional counseling if you need it. A recent study done at Stanford showed that women with breast cancer who received group therapy and lessons in self-hypnosis lived an average of almost twice as long as a similar group who had only traditional medical treatment.[121] Private counseling and a support group can work hand in hand. Together they can add to your well-being and enrich your life. But be gentle with yourself. If you do not feel able to join a group now, relax and focus on some other nurturing strategy for the time being. But please keep the option open: you may feel differently later.

My Life Has Become Unmanageable

Before we continue to the next step, there is one last concept we'd like to clarify: the second part of the first step. Some people have a hard time with this part. By now you may realize your powerlessness over being infected or at risk for infection, and the feelings that come with that. But to consider that your life has become unmanageable may cause your ego to rebel. Please keep an open mind until it makes more sense. One of Webster's definitions of *manage* is "to move or use in the manner desired." To apply this, ask yourself this question: Am I now where I had intended to be at this point in my life? If the answer is no, then you have not successfully managed your life; few of us have. This is not a matter of blame, but of fact. It is vital for you to see this so you can become willing to do things differently.

The way in which your life is unmanageable, besides being affected by HIV, is different for each person who reads this. The reasons most people have failed to manage well are related to the way they handled fear, anger, sadness, guilt, shame, and despair. Some people attempt to deal with their feelings through increased use of substances, such as alcohol, drugs, or food, or activities, such as sex, exercise, or gambling, in an attempt to dull their psychic pain. Others try to deny their feelings by looking good and staying very busy, working long hours or isolating themselves from friends and family. You may be having nightmares or anxiety attacks, or just more easily upset or quick to anger. But if you are at risk of becoming infected, or infected, your life is unmanageable owing to the feelings that come with this situation. Would any sane person manage his or her life so he or she could purposely become infected with HIV and have to endure all that represents?

Again, it doesn't matter if you became HIV infected from a blood transfusion during open heart surgery or from a dirty needle. The concept of unmanageability is important. You may be running much of your life quite well—and you're valuable and precious no matter how many parts of your life are going smoothly. But this shouldn't stop you from recognizing that HIV infection or risk thereof affects every aspect of your existence and gives everything a different slant.

Some people have to hit bottom before they turn their lives around. They can make a new start only after they suffer many, many unpleasant consequences of their behavior. This is not true for everyone. You can choose how low your bottom needs to be before you are willing to look at different ways of handling your life. Once you admit powerlessness over HIV and the subsequent emotions, and a need to manage your life differently because of them, you are ready for a new beginning. You are ready to complete your mourning of the past and pursue a new direction today.

Working Through the Emotions of the Past

As you embark on this new path, the first positive move is to free up any energy that you're spending on past history and your feelings about it. One effective way of doing this is writing about it. It is useful to write down how you think you became infected with HIV. Write out all your feelings about this. Keep in mind that there are no bad feelings, only feelings that need to be felt and expressed. Get them out on paper so you can go on. Curse and cry if you feel it will help. Allow your anger and grief to pour forth.

To deny yourself sorrow and anger is to deny yourself a natural response to some devastating facts. *This is a horrible situation!* You don't have to be brave or minimize what has happened. Now is a good time to let go of all the horrible thoughts and feelings you've been having.

Fear of Feelings

If you are afraid of your feelings, afraid that if you start crying you may never stop, you are not alone. Many of us are afraid we will lose control. But you will not go completely out of control, and you will stop crying. It may, however, take you a while to unleash all the sorrow you have stored up, so take your time. The more you let it out, the better you will feel.

Many of us were raised to ignore or hide (deny) feelings that were considered negative. As children it may not have been acceptable for us to express anger or fear. Now that you are calling your own shots, you need to give yourself permission to feel, accept, and express *all* your feelings.

Feelings are just feelings. They are inner experiences and sensations, not actions. Feeling like you want to kill someone or kill yourself does not mean you will. Most human beings have these feelings at one time or another, even if only for a split second. If every mother who *felt* like throwing her child against a wall did so, most children would be battered. You do not have to act on your feelings. It's only important that you feel them!

If you have been infected for some time you may think you have sufficiently worked through your feelings. You may want to check out how you feel right now. Try writing and see if you have any anger or grief left. You may be surprised. Many of us find that dealing with these sorts of feelings happens in layers. It's like peeling on onion. Over time we find deeper and deeper layers of our feelings. This lets us know we are continuing to heal and grow.

Try letting your tears and anger flow as you write. Beat your mattress. Scream into your pillow. Crumple up paper balls and throw them. Pound your couch. This is a hell of a predicament! Painful as it is, it is also your truth. And as much as you wish it weren't true—it is. You have every right to your feelings. Please give yourself permission to feel them. You're the only one who can give yourself this permission!

George M. tells of his and Wil G.'s first reactions. "We went home and had a long, hard cry. We were also angry at ourselves, angry for having caught this disease in the first place and for having put ourselves in this position. We felt dirty, ashamed, and afraid."[134] Mind you, we are not prescribing these feelings. Although anger, shame, and fear may be common first reactions, nobody deserves to stay with them. Keep feeling; the emotions will change, as they did for George and Wil.

You can go beyond this horrible situation. Try writing about your risk or your infection. Write how you feel about it. If you can't write, then talk, cry, scream, or shout out loud to yourself or a friend who understands your purpose. Beyond freeing up your energy, this self-expression may directly contribute to your health. A recent study demonstrated that people who wrote about painful emotional events had stronger immune systems than people who did not explore these feelings.[135]

After you have let out your anger in some safe way, try the loving light exercise described earlier in this chapter. This can help you recenter into the exhaustion and calmness that usually follow intense self-expression. Feeling exhausted indicates you have allowed yourself to feel your emotions very deeply. Congratulations. We know how hard it is.

Few people get all their feelings out in one sitting. You may want to set aside a little time each day to continue working on this cathartic process. Remain willing to face the facts and express yourself until you feel somewhat clean of your grief and anger. Feelings may resurface time and time again. When they do, you can use this first-step process to help you deal with whatever emotions are disturbing you.

First-Step Affirmations

These positive self-statements will support you in obtaining and maintaining the perspective offered by the first step. Repeat them several times a day. They will help you stay on course.

Today is the first day of the rest of my life.

Today I can maintain an attitude of honesty, open-mindedness, and willingness.

Today I can accept my HIV status and protect myself and others from further exposure to HIV and other infections.

Today, if I find myself feeling guilt, which is the past, I can bring myself back to the present moment.

Today, if I find myself feeling worry, which is the future, I can bring myself back to the present moment.

Today I can choose to stay where my power is: in the present moment, the now.

Today I can make good choices.

Today I can refrain from using any mind-altering substances.

Today, if I need help in refraining from using drugs or alcohol, I can accept that and get help.

Today I act quickly if depression comes knocking at my door. I feel the feeling and work through the grief, but I do not stay stuck in depression.

Today I work through any anger or grief that comes to me.

Today I am learning how to deeply relax my mind and body.

TWO

Mind as Healer, Mind as Slayer

STEP TWO

CAME to BELIEVE that a POWER greater than ourselves could RESTORE us to SANITY

CAME *reached a certain point or stage; arrived*

BELIEVE *to be persuaded of the truth of something*

POWER *force; strength; energy manifested in action*

RESTORE *repair; to bring back to a former and better state*

SANITY *sound; whole; healthy; having the regular exercise of reason*

Step two has three parts. First, it helps you examine how and when your thinking and acting were "insane" and may have interfered with your optimal health. Second, it acknowledges that there is a power greater than yourself that can work for you and with you. Third, it helps make plausible to you the idea that a power greater than what you have been using can help you develop a way of life that is more sane and more compatible with your optimal physical, mental, emotional, and spiritual health.

Step Two and HIV Infection

What does coming "to believe that a power greater than ourselves could restore us to sanity" have to do with HIV infection? *Sanity* refers to healthy, sound thinking. The way in which you think often determines the way you respond to situations; it can determine how you feel about a situation and how you act within it. Often our thinking is based on beliefs that we are unaware we hold. And these unconscious beliefs can direct our emotions and our behavior in ways that are not good for us. For example, we know from their own reports and also from studies that addicts have the belief deep within them that they are not enough. They unconsciously or consciously believe that they need the drug, the alcohol, the food, the person, the job, the sex, or whatever they are addicted to in order to be enough, to be okay. This belief then directs their emotions and behaviors. Louise's life is a case in point.

LOUISE'S STORY

For years Louise knew that her husband, Jerome, was an IV drug user. She was also aware that he was at risk of being infected with the AIDS virus, because he shared needles with his druggie pals. Jerome's weakness and weight loss made Louise suspect that he was infected with HIV, but Jerome would not be tested. Louise had heard that she was also at risk for becoming infected because she was Jerome's sex partner. She couldn't assert herself enough to ask him to use safe sex. She was afraid of his response and feared that he would seek sex elsewhere.

Once she had tried to bring up the subject of using condoms, but Jerome had become angry and abusive. Louise had just stopped thinking about it, and continued their relationship as always. She became depressed and despondent. The kids started "driving her crazy." Louise found herself drinking and smoking pot more and more to keep herself from worrying about the awful situation she faced each day and to help her sleep at night. She was afraid to live with, and yet afraid to live without Jerome. She was, as she put it, "trapped any way you look at it." When Louise became ill and the doctor told her that she had AIDS, she was, in a way, relieved, thinking, "It will be over soon! I'm tired of living like this."

Because HIV infection is a behavioral infection, beliefs that lead to certain behaviors put you at risk for infection and can further damage your body and hasten progression of disease. Can you see how Louise's failure to confront Jerome in regard to unsafe sex was "insane." It is not sane thinking to risk contracting a potentially fatal disease rather than upset your partner or face possible infidelity on his part. Louise did not believe she had the right to assert or protect herself. Deep inside Louise too believed she was not enough, not worthy of sticking up for herself. Louise's way of thinking contrasts with Richard's assertive stance.

RICHARD'S STORY

Richard wanted to know where he stood and what he could do about his situation. He knew he was infected as soon as he noticed the white spots in his throat. He immediately sought medical care, visiting several doctors until he found one who would work with him, not on him, or for him. He read everything he could read about the disease. He recognized what behaviors had put him at risk and stopped them to prevent further damage.

The only way Richard was able to do this was by being assertive with his old friends and not using alcohol or drugs. This was not easy, but, as Richard put it, "My life is at stake here!" He then entered counseling to work through old issues that sapped his emotional energy and found a support group that encouraged his spiritual beliefs. Six years later, Richard is glad that he did. Now he helps others do the same.

Richard's self-assertion put him in the best possible position to deal actively with his infection. We know it wasn't easy. Developing assertion skills in situations such as Louise's are sometimes extremely difficult, but you can help yourself by becoming more aware and learning to use the tools offered in this program. These tools make it easier to use sane, sound thinking, which protects you.

Additionally, how you think and how you feel influence each other, and certain feeling states are known to affect the immune system. Thus your thoughts and feelings may both affect the progression of your HIV infection. So it's important to explore any ways in which your thoughts and feelings are unhealthy, or insane, and may lead to ways of responding that have a negative impact on your emotional, spiritual, mental, and physical health. In order to be restored to sanity, it is necessary to first be aware of ways in which you are not sane, whole, and healthy.

The second step can help you tap into a power—an ability to act—greater than what you have been using. If you were able to change your life and return to sanity using your own current form of power, you would already have done so.

Came to Believe: The Magic of Belief

The wisdom of the ages points out that people who have faith, especially faith in a power greater than themselves, are able to accomplish things, heal themselves, and find fulfillment in their lives. This can also be true of people infected with or at risk of contracting HIV.

If you do not have any conscious contact with a power greater than yourself, step three will help you develop it. For now, all you have to do is be willing to accept the possible existence of some kind of Creative Intelligence or Spirit of the Universe, which underlies the totality of things.

Ask yourself, "Do I now believe or am I willing to consider the possibility that there could be a power greater than myself?" As you work through this step, try to keep yourself open to this possibility *and* the possibility that this power can restore you to sanity in the areas of your life that are presently unmanageable.

When we consider that we certainly do not cause the seasons to change or the tides to rise and fall, we may begin to recognize some kind of force that is greater and more powerful than our own. You may have watered the lawn or fertilized the plants, but it was not you who caused the grass to grow or the rose to bloom. Neither did you invent lightning, the stars, gravity or yourself. Logic would have it that there is a power greater than you and me, even though we may not yet have a clear understanding of that power.

Your Higher Power need not have a personality or take a distinct form. People who already have an understanding of a Higher Power may refer to it in various ways, such as God, the Holy Spirit, the Great Spirit, or the Universal Intelligence. For many people the Higher Power is something within themselves that guides and directs them. Some refer to this as the God Within, their own Spirit, their Higher Self, or their Soul. Others believe they have an Inner Guide or Guardian that is their Higher Power.

We are not promoting any specific religious or spiritual path. Many spiritual paths and religious paths exist, and most of them recognize the presence of a Higher Power.

Authentic Self

For those who do not relate well to the transcendent approach, there is a more secular way of interpreting this Higher Power. Think about times when you were out of control. Perhaps you had had a few drinks or taken a drug, or maybe there was a time when everything seemed to be falling apart in your life and you found yourself screaming at friends and family, doing things you would never do if you truly had your wits about you. Or perhaps you were not paying attention one day and locked your keys in your car. At that moment you were out of control. You were not centered, not working from your Higher Self.

Most of us can look back five or ten years and realize that we would not make the same choices today that we did then. What we did then may not even make much sense to us now. This shows that each of us has the potential to understand more than we seem to be able to understand. Each of us can attain a higher level of consciousness, a higher level of understanding and discernment.

One way to reach this higher level is simply to live and have many different experiences. Another way, a quicker method, is to increase our moment-by-moment awareness. When we can stay centered in the here and now, we can respond from our higher understanding and increase our ability to make wholesome choices. Thus our Higher Power can be seen as our Ideal Self, Authentic Self, or our Aware Self.

This step does not require belief. It is enough to keep an open mind regarding the idea that there may be a power greater than your own current power. When pondering this idea, imagine the possibility that this Higher Power can help you change any insane ways of thinking, feeling, or behaving. After all, the point is to maximize your well-being by aligning your beliefs, thoughts, feelings, and actions. A Higher Power can help you greatly in this quest.

Do You View the World Sanely?

Our bodies respond magnificently to positive thoughts and feelings. On the other hand, they also react to negative thoughts and feelings, which elicit the same "fight or flight" response that saved our prehistoric ancestors from tigers. This response saved our ancestors by speeding up their breathing and heart rate, and by shifting blood to their muscles, so they could run from predators to a place of safety. Now, however, we have the ability to create imaginary "tigers" in our lives.

By thinking in certain ways we keep our bodies constantly geared up for a fight or flight response, although neither fight nor flight is an effective solution to most of today's demands. Tensions and chemicals that accompany these thought patterns build up in our bodies, exhaust our energy, and leave us open to all sorts of disorders. In one study of survival times for persons with AIDS, those who were better able to deal with this fight or flight response had longer survival time.[1]

To understand how your mind rules your body, remember how your face turns red when you are embarrassed or how red can creep up the neck of a person who is speaking in public. If you even think about someone you are furious with, you can actually feel a surge of anger. Your body is already getting ready to do battle with that person. Or if you bring to mind a sad event, tears may well up in your eyes, or your stomach or chest may tighten. Again, it was only a thought, but your body does not know the difference between an event and a thought about an event. Corporations know this is true, and they spend millions of dollars every day on advertising to affect our ideas. We now know that thinking is not only an electrical event that can be measured. It is also a chemical event. How we think and feel sends various chemicals throughout our bodies.

Therefore it is critical to examine the ways in which you think, how you view the world. Are you causing yourself unnecessary stress, damaging your body in the process?

Webster defines *insane* as having "an unsound mind." Another definition we like is "repeating the same behaviors while expecting different results." Your thought habits can keep you stuck in fight or flight, fighting the same old battles in the same old ways. Step two helps you identify the ways in which your thinking is insane, or unsound. All of us think insanely sometimes; but some of us think in these ways quite often. It is in this instance that we need to make use of step two.

The Mind/Body Connection

A new medical subspecialty, psychoneuroimmunology (PNI), is devoted to studying how the mind and the body interact. Endorphins, morphinelike pain killers produced by and released from the brain during certain events, such as childbirth or jogging, were discovered in the 1970s; more than a hundred other neurotransmitters produced by the brain have since been discovered. Scientists now view the brain as a gland, a secreting organ that makes messenger chemicals that directly and indirectly influence the cells of the body, including the cells of the immune system.

The immune system is one of our defense systems, and it is designed to recognize and destroy foreign cells. It does so with a very complex set of chemicals and specialized cells, the most well-known of which are the white blood cells. There are many types of white blood cells, including B cells and T cells. Some T cells kill cancerous cells. When the immune system overreacts, or identifies its own particles as foreign particles, allergies and autoimmune diseases develop. When the immune system underreacts, infections and cancers can take hold. The mind/body connection is evident, in autoimmune disorders, such as rheumatoid arthritis and lupus. The fact that these disorders of the immune system are found more often in females and left-handed individuals indicates how dramatically hormones and the brain can influence the immune system.

Furthermore, scientists and specialists in the field of PNI are beginning to view the immune system as a floating extension of the brain. In other words, the cells of the immune system are seen as circulating nerve cells. These cells have receptors for the chemicals released by the brain and central nervous system. They are designed to receive messages directly from the brain.

The point is that perceptions and thoughts in the brain send chemical telegrams to the rest of the body. To continue the metaphor, there is a part of your brain whose function is to protect you, much as the head of the Secret Service is responsible for protecting the president. Your brain relies on these chemical messengers to activate or deactivate your immune system, much as the Secret Service chief relies on messages via telegrams or walkie-talkies to communicate with Secret Service agents. Laboratory studies show how these chemicals modulate, or give direction to, the movement of the white blood cells. Additionally, the cells themselves produce these same chemicals, pointing to a feedback mechanism from the immune system back to the brain.

Other recent developments—such as the discovery of nerves running from the brain to the thymus and lymph nodes and the discovery that activation of a certain area in the brain occurs during immune responses—vividly illustrate the interaction between the brain and the immune system. Additionally, it has been demonstrated that the immune system can actually be conditioned to suppress itself! As they contemplate the full meaning of these discoveries, PNI researchers are also looking for techniques to increase the number of health-enhancing messages sent to the cells of the immune system.

Many people believe—and there are studies to support this idea—that accepting and opening to your Higher Power is an effective way of stimulating the flow of chemicals to the immune system.

Stress and the Immune System

How stress affects the immune system is the subject of numerous studies. At the Fifth International Conference on AIDS in June 1989, one study reported that HIV-infected individuals are three times more likely to get ill when exposed to major stressor events.[2] Major stresses resulting from losses through death, surround people in the male homosexual, IV drug, and hemophiliac communities. Given such enormous strain and grief, it is even more important to learn how to cope as sanely as possible.

Given the same stressful situation, poor copers—people who have difficulty handling stress—repeatedly demonstrate a more depressed immune function than good copers—people who take stress in their stride. It is not how *much* stress you experience that determines how it will affect your body, but how you *respond* to the stress.

There are specific and nonspecific responses to stressful events. For example, for someone who is worried about whether he or she is infected with HIV, a *specific* response is to assess the risk by reviewing the ways in which people become infected with HIV. Getting tested for the antibody is another active, specific way of responding to the stress of worrying and wondering. Regardless of the test result, avoidance of high-risk behaviors is also a specific and protective response. Good copers use more specific responses that poor copers do.

Nonspecific ways of coping include worrying, having fitful sleep and nightmares, medicating anxiety with alcohol or drugs, and engaging in promiscuous sex. None of these responses really addresses the original cause of the worry. Like any nonspecific behavior, this style of coping is reactive, rather than active, and provides only temporary and false relief.

Besides impairing the immune system directly, stress also affects your DNA repair system, which is a basic line of defense against the development of cancer. DNA is the part of the chromosome that determines your inborn characteristics, such as the color of your eyes. When cells are damaged from chemicals or radiation in a person's diet or environment, it is the DNA repair system that repairs damaged genes and keeps mutations and cancerous tumors from developing.

This protective mechanism cannot work as efficiently if it is compromised by your responses to stress. Kaposi's sarcoma, KS, is one type of cancer that can develop in people infected with HIV. This is just one reason why we spend so much time in this program helping you deal with stress in a constructive way.

Depression and the Immune System

We all know that when we are depressed or anxious we are less capable of making good choices and taking care of ourselves. Additionally, it seems that depression and anxiety are especially hard on immune cells. Long-term depression places people at risk for infections and reactivation of dormant viruses. One large study showed that men whose wives had recently died were hospitalized three times more often for severe infection. You may have experienced the loss of friends or loved ones to HIV. It is important that you allow yourself to feel the feelings of grief and work through them. In step four, on page 130, is a process to help you deal with the grief of loss.

Helping Your Immune System

Other studies demonstrate that certain mind states produced by meditating, using imagery, feeling a sense of control, as well as good social support, exercise, and physical touch, help the immune cells function better. In one study a woman was able to regulate her body's response to the chicken pox virus skin test. She could change her body's response to the skin test by meditating and visualizing either a positive or a negative skin test response.

We also know that many illnesses—such as high blood pressure, coronary artery disease, migraine headaches, colitis, allergies, and asthma—are often caused by, or made worse by, our response to stressors.

As described, there are many ways to enhance and strengthen your immune system as well as just generally feel better about yourself and your place in the universe. If you are interested in the specific studies, you will find them mentioned in Chapter 15 and in the suggested reading list in the Appendix.

Attitudes and Thought Patterns

As we have discussed, certain behaviors and emotional states impair the immune system. It will be useful to look at your attitudes and thought patterns to see if any of them are affecting you and your immune system in a negative way. In order to develop attitudes and think thoughts that bolster your immune system and promote overall good health, you may need to drop certain negative attitudes and change some of your thinking patterns.

Albert Ellis, an early developer of cognitive psychotherapy, identifies ten irrational beliefs that can distort your views.[4] These thoughts result in faulty reactions and increased stress. You probably learned many of these as a child, and may continue to act on them unconsciously as an adult. These thoughts keep your body in the detrimental fight or flight response and are not sane ways of thinking. Which irrational beliefs in the following list, adapted from Albert Ellis's list, do you hold?

1. Everyone should like me.

2. I should never make mistakes.

3. Certain people or groups are always bad and deserve to be punished.

4. It is awful when things are not the way I want them to be.

5. My happiness is dependent on people, places, and things.

6. If anything bad can go wrong it will, and I may as well be prepared for it by worrying and anticipating it.

7. It is easier to avoid or not think about life's difficulties rather than face them.

8. I need to be able to depend on someone who is stronger than me.

9. My past determines my today and my response to it is unchangeable. I will continue to do as I was programmed.

10. There is a right way to do everything, and if it is not found I feel awful.

Many people base their feelings about whether they are valuable or "good" on such misbeliefs. Louise, mentioned earlier, probably held several of these misbeliefs, which kept her from being assertive with Jerome and protecting herself from infection. Many people suffer undue stress because of this faulty thinking.

You Can Challenge Your Misbeliefs

Learn to examine your misbeliefs closely, to challenge your misbeliefs. Ask yourself, "Is that *really* true, *always* true? Is that true for *this* event?" What are some other misbeliefs you hold? Write them down. Examples are, "If my spouse is unhappy, I must have done something wrong," and "If someone disagrees with me, he doesn't like me or I must be wrong."

These kinds of thoughts may be habitual and easy to slip into, but they can also be harmful. Our beliefs and distortions often operate outside our awareness, as does our immune system, so it may take some practice to tune into them as we go about our daily lives. Meanwhile, see if any of the following faulty thinking modes are ones you employ.

Global, Extreme Thinking

Global, extreme thinking has you see your experiences as very intense. Global, extreme words include, *extremely, totally, excessively, incredibly,* and *awful.*

An example might be, "I am extremely nervous." When you hear yourself using such a strong word, challenge yourself. "Really? Am I really extremely nervous?" You may find that what you actually are is somewhat nervous. Try not to exaggerate the situation.

Not many events are really awful. HIV infection is. In the beginning you may actually feel extremely upset. But if, as a rule, you use extreme thinking, and you get stuck in it, you are overstressing yourself and becoming emotionally exhausted about things that are not really awful. You then have no energy left for facing the things that may warrant such a reaction.

Absolutistic, Moralistic Thinking

Absolutistic, moralistic thinking is rigid thinking. Absolutistic, moralistic words include nobody and everybody. Often situations have nothing to do with morals. HIV infection is certainly a good example. You may have felt judged by people who are moralistic about HIV infection, and you may find yourself thinking in a moralistic way. How many times have you been certain that an issue was clearly right or wrong, black or white? If you have an open mind you'll see that most situations are a shade of gray. Listen to yourself for absolutistic thinking. It leaves you with no place to go. For example, you might think, "I can't do anything right! I am just a mess!" Change thus becomes impossible. This is not sane thinking. Change what you say to yourself. "I do many things right." [Look at your shoes: are they on the proper feet?] "Everybody makes mistakes sometimes. Just because I *made* a mistake does not mean I *am* a mistake."

Irreversible Thinking

Irreversible thinking is defeated thinking. Irreversible words include *always, never,* and *can't.* The thought that nothing can ever be done about a situation is often used as an excuse not to change behavior or to justify behavior. But this type of thinking is destructive, because it is the stance of a victim or a martyr; stances that do not allow active coping. An example is, "It's just my nature to always overreact to everything." Challenge that thought: "I used to react strongly to things, but I'm now aware that can hurt me, and I am learning how to handle things differently." Another example is, "That's just the kind of person I am." A challenge is, "Wait a minute, is that the only kind of person I am? Not really! Is it possible that I can change? Of course."

Spend some time now thinking and writing down the adjectives you use when describing an incident. Do *totally, awful, nobody, everybody, always, can't* (and similar words) show up often? Do you see a pattern? Can you imagine rewording your statements so that they are more realistic? This can help you manage and assess your stressors more easily. It can also lead to more sane thinking and responding.

Transformational Coping

Suzanne Kobasa, Ph.D., has done many studies on hardiness, looking at why certain individuals with the same level of stressors became ill while others did not.[5, 6] She found that "hardy" individuals used what she called transformational coping to deal with their problems. They used what she describes as the three Cs of hardy coping: challenge, commitment, and control. They viewed their problems as challenges, committed themselves to working through them, and sought out ways in which they could control them. Those who used this way of thinking became ill only half as often as their nonhardy counterparts.

Hardy individuals were able to stay healthy by altering their perceptions of the events so they became less stressful. They thought about them optimistically and took decisive action. Richard, discussed earlier in this chapter, is a hardy coper. He acted toward his infection in a decisive way and was able to transform it into a circumstance that generated less stress.

Members of Alcoholics Anonymous, and other twelve-step programs based on the same principles, use a simple and old prayer to help them cope with their stressful experiences. Frequent repetition of this prayer enables them to transform these events into something they can either work to change or else accept as they are.

The Serenity Prayer is as follows:

> God, grant me the serenity to accept
>   the things I cannot change,
> The courage to change the things I can,
> And the wisdom to know the difference.

Repeating this prayer is a good way to deal with your stressors. When you are in a stressful situation, just take slow, deliberate breaths (all types of meditation begin with slow, deep breathing because it is a feedback mechanism to tell the brain that all is well), and repeat the Serenity Prayer.

Is the cause of your upset something you can change? If it is, do so. If not, let it go. You can learn to turn your energy toward something you do have control over, such as your response to the situation. We realize this is a lot harder to do than it is to talk about, but we also know it works. But it takes willingness, awareness, and practice.

How to Restore Clarity and Sanity to Your Thinking

Simple slogans are another part of a twelve-step program. These can help you transform a stressful situation into an easier one. These may at first seem too simple, but there is often wisdom in simplicity. Millions of people can attest to their effectiveness! By using a simple slogan you can stop your thoughts long enough to regain clarity and defuse anxiety. You have probably seen these slogans on bumper stickers.

When you find yourself in certain troublesome ways of thinking, be gentle with yourself. This is probably a very old pattern, and it won't disappear right away. Here are specific aids that help stop this kind of thinking:

1. Stop your thought (clap your hands or say to yourself, Stop).

2. Silently thank your mind for sharing its thought.

3. Silently repeat and reflect on the meaning of one of the following slogans.

When you find yourself projecting into the future and worrying: One day at a time.

When you find yourself feeling overwhelmed and trying to do too much: Keep it simple or First things first or Turn it over (more about this last in step three) or Let go and let God.

When you find yourself in what feels like an unbearable situation or unbearable feeling and you feel like you can't get through it: It helps to remember other times in your life when something similar has happened to you and you *did* get through it.

When you find yourself becoming critical or irritated with someone: There, but for the grace of God, go I or Live and let live or Let it begin with me. Sometimes it is helpful to smile and thank your Higher Power for the opportunity to practice tolerance on another perfectly imperfect human.

This last saying is what we consider to be the most important and profound slogan. It empowers you to operate from your Higher Self and, in so doing, respond to the Higher Self of another. It is engraved on the token people in twelve-step programs are awarded on the anniversary of being sober or in the program. When you feel confused or torn between two different behaviors, one of which may be harmful: To thine own self be true. Why not write your favorite slogan on index cards or adhesive-backed notes and post them several places as reminders.

Assertiveness

Dr. George Solomon of the University of California, Los Angeles, and Lydia Temoshok, Ph.D., of the University of California, San Francisco, have been doing a study on people who developed AIDS. They have found that the people who live the longest have really only one particular quality in common: they are able to say *no* to unwanted favors. They are able to do what is in their own best interest. They are able to be true to themselves.

When you are being true to yourself, you are tapping into that part of you that is connected to your Higher Power, your Higher Self. When you do this, your Higher Self gives you the freedom and the strength to do what is in your true best interest. This freedom and strength helps you to become self-aware, cultivate a sense of responsibility toward yourself, and develop assertiveness, three qualities that are intertwined and interdependent.

Dr. Kobasa's nonhardy people—those who demonstrated twice as much illness as hardy people—used regressive coping. This coping is not sane, sound coping. Rather than acting upon events decisively, nonhardy people think about events pessimistically and act evasively to avoid contact with them. They are passive rather than assertive. To avoid illness whenever possible, you really need to be assertive in handling your stressors. In this way you too can demonstrate hardiness. Asserting your own feelings and best interests is a matter of being true to yourself.

What does it mean to be assertive? You are assertive when you stand up for your rights in such a way that the rights of others are not violated. You express your personal feelings, likes, and interests spontaneously, talk about yourself without being self-conscious, with someone openly and courteously. In studies of stress and personality styles, people who were defined as being assertive were able to avoid undue stressors, especially those related to communication and relationships. Thus they could think and act sanely.

It is especially important for you to develop assertiveness skills if you are going to adopt behavior that protects you. Like Richard, you may need to assert yourself regarding drug and alcohol use. You also need to assert yourself with your doctors and health care providers. And you need to assert yourself concerning the use of your time and energy.

Being assertive is not the same as being aggressive. Aggressive behavior denies the rights of others. It is your responsibility to be assertive to defend your own rights. Ultimately only you can do that for yourself. Any other stand allows you to play either victim or aggressor, neither of which is helpful or sane.

Here is a partial list of traditional assumptions you may have learned as a child that keep you from being an assertive adult. They are matched with a list of your actual rights. A look at this list will help you identify what to change. Put a check next to the ones you need your Higher Power or Higher Self to help you with the most.

MISTAKEN ASSUMPTIONS	LEGITIMATE RIGHTS
1. It is selfish to put my needs ahead of others' needs.	1. Sometimes I have a right to put myself first.
2. It is shameful to make mistakes. I should have an appropriate response for every occasion.	2. I have a right to make mistakes. Every human being makes mistakes.
3. If I can't convince others that my feelings are reasonable, then they must be wrong, or maybe I am going crazy.	3. I have a right to be the final judge of my feelings and accept them as legitimate.
4. I should respect the views of others, especially if they are in a position of authority. I should keep my differences of opinion to myself and simply listen and learn.	4. I have a right to have my own opinions and convictions.

MISTAKEN ASSUMPTIONS	LEGITIMATE RIGHTS
5. I should always be logical and consistent.	5. I have a right to change my mind, to decide on a different course of action.
6. I should never interrupt people. Asking questions reveals my stupidity.	6. I have a right and a responsibility to politely interrupt in order to seek clarification.
7. Things could get even worse. Don't rock the boat.	7. I have a right to negotiate for change.
8. I shouldn't take up others' valuable time with my problems.	8. I have a right to ask for help or emotional support.
9. People don't want to hear that I feel badly, so I keep it to myself.	9. I have a right to feel and express pain.
10. If someone takes the time to give me advice, I should take it seriously. Others are usually right.	10. I have a right to ignore the advice of others.
11. I should always try to accommodate others. If I don't, they won't be there when I need them.	11. Sometimes I have a right to put myself first.
12. I should never refuse to socialize with others. People are going to think I don't like them if I say I'd rather be alone instead of being with them.	12. I have a right to be alone, even if others would prefer my company.
13. I should always have a good reason for what I feel and do.	13. I have a right not to have to justify myself to others all the time.
14. When someone is in trouble, I should always help him or her.	14. I have a right not to take responsibility for someone else's problems.
15. I should always be sensitive to the needs and wishes of others, even when they are unable to tell me what they want.	15. I have a right not to have to anticipate others' needs and wishes.
16. It's not nice to put people off. If questioned, I should give an answer.	16. I have a right to choose not to respond to a situation.

Assertiveness and Women

The majority of women infected with HIV are IV drug addicts, or sex partners of infected men. The majority are women of color, from black or Hispanic cultures. If you are a woman of color, it may be very hard for you to be assertive with your sex partners, owing to cultural messages that the man is in charge. It may also be very hard for you to stop using drugs. Learning assertion skills will help you in both areas.

You may feel financially or emotionally dependent on your partner and even fear physical abuse if you try to negotiate safe sex. This is certainly a tough position to find yourself in, but as you probably know, almost every baby infected with the AIDS virus is the baby of a black or Hispanic woman who is either addicted to drugs or having unsafe sex with an HIV-infected man.

Whether you are the wife of a hemophiliac, partner of an IV drug user, or a woman who is sexually active and dating, it is equally important that you protect yourself sexually. Although not many men who are not in high-risk groups are infected, some are. It is easier to transmit the virus from man to woman than from woman to man. And even though not all partners of HIV-positive men become infected, many do.

This is not a sexually trasmitted disease that a dose of penicillin will cure. This is the kind of exposure no one can afford. You must act assertively to protect yourself, even if the thought of buying condoms is repulsive to you. Remember that this is not for birth control purposes, so if you use some other method of birth control, you still need to use condoms to prevent infection. And even if you are already pregnant you will need to use condoms to protect you and the fetus from further infection.

These are things you need to know. By being assertive regarding high-risk sexual behavior, you protect not only yourself from infection, but also your unborn infants. We know you would never want anything to happen to your babies. If you are already infected the virus can be in your milk, so it is important that you *not* breast feed.

If you are a member of a minority, get help from someone who understands your culture. Many cities have outreach workers who are recovering addicts. They can explain things in such a way that your partner can understand and learn to protect himself and you. If he won't listen, these people can help you learn how to be assertive about sex so you can protect yourself. They have fliers that can give you ideas on how to approach your partner. Or if you have to leave to protect yourself and your babies while you are still healthy, they can help you do it. We wish there were another way, but if your partner is at risk for infection, so are you and your unborn children! If you are doing IV drugs, you already know you must find a way to stop.

Positive Self-Talk: Being True to Myself

In addition to posting slogans, you may want to find ways to remind yourself of these affirmations as you work through this second step.

- I know that prolonged depression and anxiety can be harmful to my immune system.

- I am learning new ways to deal with my feelings so I can avoid depression and needless anxiety.

- I am able to transform my anxieties by using the Serenity Prayer and some simple slogans.

- I concentrate on the things that I can change.

- I find ways to accept things that I cannot change.

- I am learning to live one day at a time.

- I practice my relaxation processes daily.

- If I feel stressed, I stop, take deep breaths, and bring my healing light into my body to calm me.

- I want to be assertive so I can protect myself from unnecessary stress, unsafe sex, alcohol use, drug abuse, and worry.

- I am becoming a hardy coper by transforming my response to stressors.

- I change my thinking and change my response to stressors in my daily living in a way that serves me.

Induced, Frozen, and Carried Feeling States

Pia Mellody, R.N., works with people with addictions and histories of childhood abuse. She describes certain other problems concerning feelings in her book *Facing Codependence.*[7] We believe her descriptions are accurate. She says that people who have been abused in any way have trouble experiencing their feelings in moderation. They feel either little or no emotion or else experience explosive, almost overwhelming emotions. This happens because of certain types of feelings:

1. *Induced feelings* are feelings that you absorb from another person. You may take on the other's feelings either because they are very intense or because the other person is denying the feelings. Can you remember when someone else was very angry, sad, or bitter, and suddenly your good mood shifted to one of anger, sadness, or bitterness. You absorbed the other's feeling. Or can you think of the last time someone you knew was very angry, but wouldn't talk about it and told you that he or she was fine. Did you then become so angry that you felt almost crazy? These absorbed feelings leave you feeling crazy because they do not make sense to you. They do not make sense to you because they are not your feelings!

   When you are with someone and find yourself suddenly feeling crazy, stop and ask yourself, "When did I start feeling like this?" If it started when you were with that other person, check to see if you absorbed his or her feelings. Then, if appropriate, tell yourself that is what happened and brush off your shoulders. Imagine you are brushing off those feelings like you brush off dandruff or spider webs. Or take a shower and imagine the feelings going down the drain. Take deep breaths and repeat an affirmation, such as, "I'm getting calmer. I'm letting go of the feelings; they don't belong to me and I don't want them! I feel better already. They're almost gone."

2. *Frozen feelings* are feelings that "froze" within you when you were a child. Usually frozen feelings are anger, pain, or fear. These feelings can start to "thaw" and leak out when something triggers them. When they do, which is healing, you may feel very small, vulnerable, and childlike. Have you ever found tears

coming when you watched a mushy movie, or gotten hysterical when you thought someone you loved was going to leave you?

Many of us were abandoned in many ways when we were very little. We were abandoned by our parents in favor of work, another person, or an addiction. Or we were emotionally abandoned through abuse. Back then our very survival depended on that other person being there. But now as adults, if that childhood fear starts to thaw when we think another adult is leaving we might react and really feel like our very survival depended on his or her staying. When that happens do you feel very little and afraid, and maybe even sound like a child? That is your childhood fear being triggered. Try to be gentle with yourself, feeling that the feeling is healing, although incredibly painful. This is the time to let that little person who lives inside you know that it is okay to feel the feeling and that you are not going to leave! Then try to remember other times when you felt like this and remember that you did live through it. You *can* make it and you *will* make it!

3. *Carried feelings* are feelings you absorbed as a child from someone who abused you. These are usually feelings of shame that the abuser should have had, but did not feel himself or herself. Like a little sponge, you absorbed your abuser's shame. When you have carried feelings it is a feeling of being overwhelmed and out of control over a relatively simple incident. These are called shame attacks, and come from feelings carried since childhood.

Have you ever felt like you wanted to die, run away, or hit someone when he or she mildly criticized you? Ask yourself what the feeling reminds you of. If you can, write about it. You may be surprised at what you find out about your childhood. Writing somehow unlocks a part of your mind that otherwise often stays closed. If you can't write, just say to yourself, "This reminds me of that-was-then/this-is-now. Today I know I'm not perfect. I am a perfectly imperfect human being, just the way my Higher Power made me. In the grand scheme of things, this is not a big deal. I'm still precious and I know it. I will live through this!"

Unfortunately, these absorbed, frozen, and carried feelings can make you feel really crazy. But it is important to remember that *feeling* crazy doesn't mean you *are* crazy! And anyone who has been abused has these kinds of feelings. Knowing where they come from helps, and therapy with someone who does inner child work is very valuable.

Insane Behaviors

You also need to look at any behaviors that place you at a greater risk to develop or hasten the disease process. Keep in mind that *HIV infection is a behavioral infection.* In other words, if you do not engage in activities that transmit the virus, you will not become infected.

Unfortunately, many people were infected with HIV before it was known that they were at risk. The blood pool was contaminated with HIV and distributed before it was known to be contaminated. Therefore, many hemophiliacs who received blood concentrates were infected. Their behavior that permitted the infection was not known to be a risk and was intended to preserve their lives, not endanger them. People who received contaminated blood transfusions, who were inseminated with infected semen, or who received infected organs were likewise infected.

In the first few years of the epidemic it was not clear exactly how the disease was transmitted. Therefore thousands of people were infected by activities that were not considered then to be high-risk behaviors. By the time we knew how the disease was transmitted, many people were already unknowingly infected. But now we do know, and now you have choices that others didn't. The behaviors we are about to discuss can not only give you the infection, but can make your illness worse, as well as transmit it to others.

High-Risk Behaviors

You may be aware of what behaviors are risky, but we will list them for review again. *Behaviors that spread HIV infection include*

- the sharing of needles or syringes

- anal sex (with or without a condom, because of frequent condom breakage and minuscule rectal abrasions)

- unprotected vaginal or oral sex with someone who shoots drugs or engages in anal sex
- unprotected vaginal or oral sex with someone whose risk is unknown to you
- unprotected vaginal or oral sex with an infected person
- the sharing of sex toys

Protected sex refers to using a *latex* condom that has an inner coating of *nonoxynol-9* or using a *latex* condom along with a cream, foam, or gel that contains nonoxynol-9 and *only* a water-soluble lubricant (such as KY jelly) for intercourse. Vaseline, lotions, and oils are *not* water soluble and cause condom breakage.

Cofactors

Your risk of becoming infected or aggravating your infection increases with each cofactor. Chapter 1 discusses cofactors at length. We bring up two cofactors again to reiterate their risks.

Sexual Cofactors as Insane Behaviors

Any sexually transmitted disease increases the number of white blood cells in the genital area. The AIDS virus lives and multiplies in these white blood cells. And skin sores from these sexually transmitted diseases allow easy entry for the AIDS virus. This may be the reason people who have other sexually transmitted diseases become more easily infected with HIV. In a recent study, two factors linked to HIV disease progression were the number of sexual partners and the number of sexually transmitted diseases a person had.

If you were infected through a transfusion, artificial insemination, or an infected transplanted organ, do not ignore this section. You may not participate in some of these high-risk behaviors, but you can still infect people sexually. In fact, many people infected from transfusions are *not* protecting their sex partners! The Centers for Disease Control report that 75 percent of the women who have become infected from unprotected sex became so from sexual partners who showed no signs of illness. More and more sexual partners of hemophiliacs are becoming infected. If you or your partner have not become infected yet, it does not mean that you won't. People with the virus seem to become more contagious as time goes on.

Many sex partners of hemophiliacs refuse to be tested. The problem with not being tested is the risk to the woman and the baby if she becomes pregnant. About 10 percent of pregnant wives of hemophiliacs who permitted testing turned out to be infected with the virus. Approximately 50 percent of those babies will be born infected. So the not knowing, and the refusal to have safe sex, have now put these unborn children as well as the mothers in mortal danger. The National Hemophilia Foundation published a medical bulletin (#76) on Feb. 14, 1989, entitled "Urgent Need to Monitor HIV Infection and Your Immune System," telling sexual partners of hemophiliacs who received blood products before 1985 to get tested for the HIV antibody. The bulletin went on to say that any partner who tested positive should have immune system monitoring every three to six months, as well as suggested treatment protocols.

Drug and Alcohol Cofactors as Insane Behaviors

If using drugs or alcohol led you to engage in behaviors that may have endangered your health and well-being, you need to accept that so you can now make saner choices.

We know that HIV can infect the brain and cause many psychological disturbances. But people who continue to use drugs or alcohol are reported to exhibit *five times* more psychiatric disorders than other infected individuals. This is one more important reason to discontinue using any mind-altering substances.

Review your drug and alcohol use, and look at ways this use affected your thinking and led you to think, feel, and act in insane ways. Write about the times when you became physically sick from substance abuse, the times when you endangered your own or someone else's life (such as when driving under the influence), and the times when your behavior was not that of your Higher Self. Did you lose any friends or damage any relationships owing to substance abuse? Were you dishonest as a result of, or to cover up, your drug or alcohol use? Can you remember hangovers, "crashing," hallucinations, paranoia, fear, anger, desperation, guilt, shame, or any other negative feeling?

The more honestly, openly, and willingly you set about this, the longer your list may be. The point is not to condemn yourself, but to create a realistic picture of your past that helps you shed a habit. Drugs and alcohol are not easy to leave behind, so the longer the list, the better. You can use it to help yourself.

Aside from what you list, you have an even more urgent reason to stop using alcohol or drugs. Now you know that even occasional use is contrary to your best interests. As we said before, alcohol and drugs somehow actually make the HIV infection worse. Can you see how insane it would be to continue abusing alcohol or using drugs? Whatever risk group, or combination of risk groups, you may be in, you need to look at your behaviors, accept responsibility for your actions, and give yourself a new way of life, that is healthier, more centered, and more joyful.

Start by making a list of the insane behaviors that you want to change. See them clearly on paper. Picture yourself doing things differently. You *can* change. The male homosexual and bisexual communities have set very good examples regarding change. Now that they know what sexual behaviors put them at high risk, most have changed accordingly. The rate of sexually transmitted disease in homosexuals and bisexuals has dropped significantly, but the rate for heterosexuals is rising!

You can change too. All you need do is remain open, remain willing to allow a power greater than yourself to restore you to sanity. You are doing a great job in making changes. The fact that you are reading this book and following these processes means that you are making a sincere effort. Good for you!

Spiritual Attunement Imagery

The following imagery process will help you experience your Higher Power and allow it to help create balance and wholeness in your body, emotions, and mind. Use this imagery process frequently, at least once a day. Be patient. Soon you will begin to feel your Higher Power working daily in your life. Relax with the deep relaxation from Chapter 1 on page 38. For a more complete script, see page 282 in appendix.

Part 1: Deep Relaxation

Before you start, eliminate any possibility of interruption or distraction so that you can focus completely upon relaxation, peace, and your own healing. Unplug the phone, put a sign on the door, let people know that you are going to be taking some time for your own healing and unstressing. Loosen any constricting clothing and sit or lie in a comfortable position.

Part 2: Tuning to the Spirit

Take a deep breath in, and as you let the air out, allow your mind to clear itself of all thoughts, images, and words. As you breathe, imagine yourself floating within a bubble of crystal light. Imagine you are traveling to the very essence of your being.

Imagine that here in the center of the silence is a Presence beyond naming, whom you might refer to as God or Love or Universal Wisdom or perhaps the Life Force, your Higher Power. Imagine that you can look forward through time and see yourself developing, healing, gaining more and more wisdom and becoming more whole. Now imagine that you are that more developed person, right here, right now.

Picture your body as healthy, whole, comfortable, vigorous, and energetic. See yourself doing anything you'd really like to be doing. See yourself as you'd really like to be. With each breath, breathe energy from this image into your physical body. Picture your body being transformed into this image.

With each exhalation repeat one of the following statements, changing any words to make it even *more* true for you. Work your way through the list, repeating the list as often as you'd like.

I am not my body.

I am not my mind.

I am not my emotions.

I see beyond the world of the senses.

This moment is the only moment there is.

Only my body exists in time.

I realize all that is physical will pass away.

I am not attached to the physical world.

I am guided by an inner experience of light, peace, joy, and love.

My spirit is a light that dispels darkness and fear.

I have learned the freedom that comes with forgiveness.

I guide all forces internal and external toward their greatest good.

I allow love to flow through me.

My Higher Power works through my spirit, and I heal my mind, my body, and my spirit.

Part 3: Reawakening

Gently reorient yourself to the physical world around you, moving your arms and legs. If you wish you may instead drift into a restful slumber.

Second-Step Affirmations

The following positive self-statements will help you realize the benefits of the second step.

Today is the first day of the rest of my life.

Today I realize that I cannot use old behaviors and expect new results.

Today I challenge any old misbeliefs that stand in the way of my healing.

Today I put into my body and mind only things that nourish my body and mind.

Today I use only safe sex and avoid all drug and alcohol use.

Today I am willing to explore the concept of a Higher Power.

Today I am willing to believe that my Higher Power can restore me to sanity.

Today my Inner Healer is alive and well.

THREE

Awakening The Healer Within

STEP THREE
Made a DECISION to TURN our WILLS
and our lives OVER to the CARE OF GOD
as we UNDERSTAND GOD

DECISION *choice; final judgment or opinion*

TURN OVER *to put into different hands;
to transfer*

WILL *power or control that the mind possesses
over its own operations*

CARE OF *watchful regard and attention; concern
for safety*

GOD *Higher Power; any positive force you believe
to be more powerful than yourself*

UNDERSTAND *to apprehend or comprehend fully;
to know the meaning of*

The first action in step three is making a decision. If you have not yet developed a concept of a personal Higher Power, this step will help you do that. Additionally, you learn how turning your will and your life over to this Higher Power lightens the burden of HIV infection and enhances your total healing.

The Third Step and HIV Infection

HIV infection and AIDS are probably the major global tragedies of the twentieth century. They are horrible reminders that
throughout history human beings have endured tragic and almost
unbelievable emotional, mental, and physical pain. In turn, past
tragedies show us something survivors have in common. Whether
it be those whom Viktor Frankl discusses in his work about the
concentration camps of World War II[1] or the more recent Vietnam
prisoners of war, survivors say they were able to withstand such
hellish conditions because they had a spiritual, nonphysical connection that kept them going. By linking up with a Source of Power
greater than they or their captors possessed, they were enabled
to transcend their physical and mental torture and even their
emotional pain. They found purpose, held on and kept going when
things looked very bleak. They all comment that without this
thread of hope, faith, and a sense of purpose, they would not have
made it. They really utilized the concept of "This too shall pass."

The third step challenges us to develop a connection, a sense
of spirit, a link to a Force greater than ourselves and greater than
any man or woman. Step three shows you how to turn your
problems and fears over to that Power. Once you are connected to
this ultimate source of Power, you can relax your unnecessary
worrying, your frantic overdoing, your anxiety, and your sense of
burden. You can let this Force take over by "turning it over." In
this way, when you personally feel weak or overpowered by life or
the many events related to HIV infection, you can give your
problems over to an all-powerful, all-wise Force that can sustain
you and grapple with your problems while you regain your much-
needed strength.

MICKEY'S STORY

*Mickey became ill again, like so many times before, but
somehow this was different; he couldn't even get himself out
of bed to go "score." He finally went to the clinic and was
told he had AIDS. Devastated, Mickey cursed the Higher
Power he didn't believe in and refused to do anything his*

doctor suggested. He spent his time conning people into bringing him drugs, feeling sorry for himself, and constantly cursing "the son of a bitch who gave me the sickness." In the process he "used up" his family and real friends, emotionally, financially, and spiritually.

Only his younger sister, Theresa, would still speak to him. When she suggested that he listen to what the doctor said, Mickey replied, "What the hell does he know?" She tried everything she could imagine to get him into a better mood. She tried to get him to talk to the parish priest, a friend of the family. Mickey responded with pure bitterness and spite. She even asked him to at least say some prayers with her. "You expect me to pray to some kind of God that would let me get this goddamned sick!" he shouted. He had been unable and unwilling to accept any responsibility for his life before his infection and this attitude remained. Mickey died the way he had lived: alone and poisoned with hatred for himself and others.

Whenever we're confronted with a challenge, a crisis, or a tragedy, we have to make a choice. How will we respond? Or will we just react? We can attempt to deny, to make a choice to merely defend ourselves—or we can attempt to make a useful choice.

Mickey had the opportunity to choose, and he chose merely to react. He denied for years, and then when he could deny no longer, he chose to simply defend his angry, resentful, cynical view of the world. But he could have made a creative choice. He could have chosen to grow spiritually, to use his remaining weeks, months, or years to learn more about himself and others, and to discover the meaning and purpose of his life.

Had he done so, the change in attitude may have improved his health, and, along with changing his health habits, it may have actually kept him alive longer. And if he had gone on to die, he might have died with a feeling of serenity, with a faith in something greater than his own individual life, and in the knowledge that he could love and be loved.

For the Nonbeliever

To some it is self-evident that there is a Universal Wisdom far greater than our limited intelligence. You don't have to hold a religious belief to accept that there is quite clearly an Intelligence far greater than your own. The digestive system is a perfect example. Each day we eat our meals, some days enjoying the experience of eating more than others. We eat and pay no further attention to the food we just placed in our bodies. Somehow that food is then digested, absorbed, and converted into usable substances. These are then used by the various cells to produce muscle, bone, blood, and all the other tissues of our bodies. Simultaneously, through digestion, energy is produced to maintain the process of digestion itself, among many other processes. This is the same energy that sustains our very lives. Furthermore, minerals, vitamins, and electrolytes are being measured, and this information is fed back to specific organs. That which is needed is absorbed by our bodies; that which is not needed is eliminated.

This is just a small example of the many complex activities our bodies do each day, day in and day out. We never stop to think whether our kidneys measured the proper amount of sodium and water and properly disposed of the rest. We know that we eat and we know that we eliminate our waste products, but most of us really don't have a clue as to the nature of what happens in between. Our bodies take care of the rest automatically. Clearly, there is an Intelligence at work within each of us that is beyond our understanding, one that continues to operate for us, without our direction, at all times.

The Magic of "As If"

For now, you may have to act "as if" regarding your Higher Power. An ancient Christian saying about faith is, "Act as if you have faith, and faith will be given you." Similar phrases heard often in other twelve-step programs are "Act 'as if'" and "Fake it till you make it." These are useful when trying out new ideas or behaviors that do not yet feel comfortable.

If you are like the rest of us, you have acted "as if" many times in your life. In new jobs you probably did not feel totally qualified at first. Nevertheless, you probably pretended to act confident, all the while working your brain overtime to figure out the system. In time you *did* figure it out and *then* you had confidence. At this point you were no longer pretending. Perhaps you've walked into a roomful of strangers and acted as if you belonged. It was only after you met someone you could relate to that you really felt comfortable and as if you fit in. You acted "as if" in the beginning. We all do it every day; we're so used to doing it that we don't realize that we are "faking it till me make it" on a regular basis.

In the beginning, consciously acting "as if" may feel awkward, so please keep an open mind. Try to become like a little child for whom all things are possible. Suspend your criticism and withhold your judgment. In the beginning, pretend as long as you need to. If any other part of this program is uncomfortable for you, acting "as if" can help you until you have a clearer understanding and your comfort level improves. You may need to say to yourself, I don't know if all this affirmation and prayer stuff really works, but I'll give it a shot and act "as if" I believe it will. Just "fake it till you make it." Eventually you will feel more comfortable with the program.

When we say "*act* as if," understand that we do *not* mean "*feel* as if." Never deny your feelings. Remember, all feelings need to be felt and dealt with, so they don't get trapped inside and get acted out in oblique ways. That's why we strongly suggest you find a buddy, sponsor, or counselor to help you explore your feelings. Many people are distanced from their feelings, so dealing with them may be new. When it comes to new ways of thinking and acting, you may need to "*act* as if," but never "*feel* as if."

Developing a positive attitude and acting "as if" will also enhance your medical treatments and help you in many other respects. All things are endured best with a positive attitude, and HIV infection is no exception. But remember that everything you learn in this program is to be done *along with*, not instead of, your medical program.

What this Step Is Not

We are in no way suggesting that you have to suddenly become religious. You don't need to see this Higher Power as divine or supernatural. If you practice a religion that is of comfort to you, wonderful. But you do not need to become involved in an organized religion. You may choose to believe that this Source of Power originates in nature, the spirit of humanity, or any universal force that you can relate to as being a more powerful resource, one stronger than yourself. Some people in Alcoholics Anonymous use the AA group as their Higher Power until they can find something more personal. Surely any group of people working together and supporting each other has more power than the individual, so if you want to use your support group as your Higher Power, that will work just fine.

What this Third Step Is

There is a unique meaning to the phrases "turn it over" and "surrender" in the context of the third step. These phrases are not cop-outs, are not meaningless magical thinking, and do not mean giving up, becoming helpless or hopeless. And they do not mean doing nothing and expecting results. You are very busy doing the footwork, making real efforts to change your life. It is you who are reading this page and you who are doing the relaxation processes, getting social support, and doing the suggested writing that accompanies the steps. It is you who are doing the affirmations, you who are following whatever medical regime you are on, you who are changing your behavior and attitudes to ensure your maximum health. This is all your part. But you then need to turn the outcome over to a Power greater than yourself. Only in this way can you have any sense of peace and comfort.

Mahatma Gandhi paraphrased the Bhagavad Gita in part: "Do not identify with the actor. Do not identify with the fruits of the action. Full effort is full victory." In other words, the victory is *now!* If you are doing all the things that you can do now, that's *all* you need do. The victory *has already been won.* This is the attitude that brings about victory. Focusing on what you can do right now works much better than constantly worrying and struggling to try to make something happen. We will cover this in more detail as we go along.

"This too Shall Pass"

It is said that the biblical King Solomon had bouts of deep depression. Sometimes for days on end he felt despondent. All things around him looked dreary and he became incapable of making intelligent decisions. And if he was like most people who get depressed, he probably had either difficulty sleeping or slept far too much, didn't eat right, and didn't exercise.

Finally King Solomon summoned the wisest of his advisers and commanded him to find him some relief from this periodic pain of depression. Dutifully the wise man agreed to undertake this seemingly impossible task. He returned weeks later, carrying with him a ring. He bade King Solomon to put on the ring. "Each time you feel depressed, simply look down at the ring," he told the king. Looking at the ring, King Solomon saw an inscription: "This too shall pass."

From that point on, whenever King Solomon's spirits sank he looked at his ring and pondered the meaning of the phrase inscribed thereon. And it is said that his spirits did not ever sink as far again, nor did his depressions last as long. Many great sages throughout the ages have reminded us that in times of great pain as well as times of great joy, "This too shall pass." Remembering this is crucial to maintaining internal balance, which, in turn, is essential to health and healing.

Flowing with and Through Depression

In addition to dealing with your own HIV status, you may be experiencing one loss after another. Many of your friends may be dying. And others may not be able to cope with your new circumstances and may have left your life. If you are dealing with major behavior changes, there are many losses attached to that, such as the loss of old comforts from alcohol and drugs. This may be an entirely new way of life for you, and at times you may feel very frustrated and upset. You may be experiencing loss of a job, loss of relationships, loss of financial security, not to mention the physical challenges or limitations and the discomfort involved in some treatments.

This disease has tragedy built in at every turn, so *please* be gentle with yourself and honor your losses. They are very real. You deserve to feel your pain and not allow anyone to minimize it. But please don't feel this pain alone! Use your support systems. Go to twelve-step meetings and groups. Talk with your friends, family, sponsors, and counselors. Cry, rip paper, beat your mattress. Feel your feelings. You deserve to honor yourself in that way. Get your feelings out so they don't get stuck and end up exploding into uncontrollable rage or imploding into depression. They are your feelings, and you need to allow yourself to feel them.

On a day-to-day basis, when you are living life on life's terms and feeling fear or not feeling physically well, it is very easy to get caught up in self-pity and depression. That is different from feeling your feelings. Rather than "letting the feeling run you," you need to "run the feeling" or at least "flow with the feeling." Acknowledge it, accept it, and work through it. Call a friend or write about the feeling or the concepts discussed in the First Step, rather than get lost in depression.

Some people who find that they easily become depressed actually set a time limit on self-pity and depression. They may, for example, silently say, "All right, I'm really feeling depressed right now. I'm going to give myself until 6 P.M. to just feel good and sorry for myself. Then I'm going to go for a walk or watch TV or draw a picture or listen to a tape: anything to break the pattern of depression." This method becomes easier with practice.

One expression used in behavioral psychology really works: "Move your muscles; change your thoughts." This works whether your thoughts and feelings are about depression or pain or addictive cravings. Your mind can stay focused in only one place at a time, so engaging in some activity can replace the harmful thought.

It is very normal to have feelings of depression, but prolonged depression is especially dangerous and can interfere with your caring for yourself in many ways. Depression impairs the cells of your immune system. Therefore, if you have or are at risk of developing HIV infection, it is important that you find a way out of prolonged self-pity and depression. Certain individuals, under careful observation by a physician, may benefit from antidepressant drugs. Psychoactive drugs, however, are somewhat unpredictable, especially in HIV-infected individuals and people with substance abuse problems. Therefore, this needs close monitoring by a physician very familiar with HIV infection, psychoactive drugs, and substance abuse, if these are the issues. Another surefire way to reverse depression is to change your focus and develop what twelve-step programs refer to as an attitude of gratitude. The following exemplifies this attitude.

Not Taking Your Body for Granted

Turning your will and your life over to the Higher Power of your understanding means trusting that Higher Power. Part of trusting that Higher Power means acknowledging the extraordinary gifts you have received. One such gift is your body. You don't like to be taken for granted and neither does your body.

A folk story comes to mind about a proud moose. The source of his great pride was his marvelous spreading antlers, but he was embarrassed about his legs, which he considered spindly. He could often be seen holding his magnificent antlers high in the setting sun, but was always careful to stand in the tall weeds to hide his legs.

One day some hunters with their dogs suddenly appeared and took chase. The moose couldn't run away because his antlers got caught in the tree branches, and his strong legs couldn't carry him away from the hunters. He was shot. As he lay bleeding to death, he thought of what a fool he had been. His magnificent antlers had led to his capture by preventing his spindly but powerful legs from carrying him to safety. We too often take for granted that which serves us best.

Thankfulness

- When I focus on the millions of cells and numerous organs that are presently doing a marvelous job in my body, I can keep in touch with my Higher Power, which orchestrates it all.

- This positive way of focusing helps me keep my perspective and avoid depression.

- My Inner Healer has been operating throughout my entire lifetime.

- I no longer choose to take my miraculous body for granted.

- Today I choose to work hand in hand with my Inner Healer for the good of all of me.

- I spend time each and every day thanking some of the parts of my body for their continued dedication to my health and healing, and I do my part to participate in that miracle.

Healing

The English word *heal* comes from an Anglo-Saxon root that means "whole, hale, and hearty." Your Inner Healer is the keeper of your wholeness. Every second it is constantly breaking down and building up your body, maintaining homeostatis, or balance. We must go beyond the Hollywood-inspired, simplistic view that healing means suddenly throwing away your crutches and walking off into the sunset. Healing means the development of wholeness, gaining or regaining full function, full power, and the ability to express your unique potential, physically, emotionally, spiritually, and intellectually.

The body falls away from each of us eventually. A curious discovery is that many people find themselves healed in other ways when their physical form is at its weakest, when they are seriously or terminally ill. They find an emotional, spiritual, and intellectual healing that surpasses all understanding.

LEE'S STORY

Lee was the sponsor of coauthor Cindy Miluscak-Cooper, her guide and confidante. At the age of sixty-seven Lee came to terms with her homosexuality. She had been raised to believe that homosexuality was a mortal sin and had lived with her shame for more than forty years; she had believed that deep in her core she was bad, full of sin, and deserved punishment.

It was only because of repeated difficulty in relationships that Lee sought counseling. She was finally able to work through these agonizing issues with a therapist who was a recovering alcoholic priest who was also gay.

Cindy did not consciously know that Lee was homosexual when she asked her to be her sponsor. Lee had been sexually inactive for more than eighteen years and had never discussed her past with anyone. She was so filled with self-loathing that she did not believe anyone could love her if he or she knew. She was advised by her therapist to first disclose her sexual orientation to someone she could trust. She was told that it was this secret that caused her lack of self-acceptance and interfered with her developing healthy relationships.

Lee chose to tell Cindy. Cindy felt privileged that Lee could trust her in this very personal way, and reassured her that she had loved her and respected her before and now respected her even more because of her immense courage.

After many therapy sessions Lee would be upset and complain, "Cindy, I just can't do this. Father says that I need to learn to accept and love myself. He wants me to forgive myself! How can I? I still think it is a sin! I'm too old to change my thinking. I wish I had never started this damn counseling!"

But Lee was not too old to change her thinking—and she was not too old to start loving and accepting herself. After much emotional agony, she was finally able to feel at peace in her heart about her sexuality. She started going to gay twelve-step meetings and remained loved and accepted in the hetero-sexual community. She chose to remain celibate, but now it was a choice, not owing to shame.

As Lee would tell it, "Well, honey, I guess this is just how God made me. Who am I to criticize his handiwork? I feel so good, like a monkey has been lifted off my back. I feel as if I've been reborn. I don't think I ever really loved or accepted me before, never in my entire life!"

Lee developed a potentially terminal illness one week later. Her response was one of adaptive denial and anger. She vented this anger on her closest friends, especially when they questioned her faith in her doctor's decisions. She would then withdraw. She had long periods of extreme peace and serenity, but at times became easily frustrated. Her physical condition deteriorated very rapidly, and she required two major operations within one month. Failing to heal from them, she became stoically resigned, sharing her intimate concerns with only her closest friends, who accepted her feelings and thoughts and did not try to change her perception of reality. Cindy, being a nurse of critically ill patients for years, was probably the person closest to her through this part of her illness and felt Lee was ready to let go of the body she felt she could no longer trust. It seemed as if her last major challenge was over; she seemed almost eager for the rest and comfort she felt awaited her. She made out a living will and asked Cindy to be responsible for her medical decisions. Lee had been raised in an orphanage and had no family. At the end of her life she had a family of choice. Cindy was the daughter she had never had, and Cindy's girls were the grandchildren she had never had.

Because Lee had lived her life for so many years by the twelve steps, she had no unfinished business. The last area that had needed healing had been the lesbian issue, and it had been totally healed. She had no fear of dying and was able to talk freely about her feelings toward her intense suffering and impending death. With nothing left to fear and no more secrets, she had a miraculous healing: Lee healed into death.

Touching the Source

So, then, you may ask as you contemplate your Inner Healer, what is the role of medicine? What about the wonder drugs and the miracles of modern surgery? Are these not the real healers? The surgeon may take out the infected appendix, but your body heals the wound. The antibiotic may weaken the bacteria, but it is ultimately your body that destroys and eliminates them. What remarkable accomplishments! What Force, what Source of energy and wisdom, keeps this miraculous body of yours operating and repairing itself? Whatever you choose to call it, it has certainly served you well over the years. But even though this Inner Healer is always there, your behavior can either support or block its positive effects.

Experience and research show that you do have a Power or Inner Healer available to you that you can tap into any time you desire. All you have to do is acknowledge its presence. Some people do so through prayer, others through meditation, self-talk, or affirmations. *How* you do it is not important. *That* you *do* it *is* important. You can find unexpected strength and calm when you turn your will and your life over to the care of God as you understand God.

Time Out

Sometimes we just need to turn away from the problem at hand for the solution to come to us. Often we are standing so close that we can't see the forest for the trees. Albert Einstein said that when he was stumped over a problem he would just put it into his mind, affirming that he would get the answer, and go to sleep. In a dream the answer would come. Many artists, writers, and others find that the answer comes to them not when they struggle, but when they "turn it over."

Continuously worrying about a situation for which no solution is immediately apparent only makes the situation look worse. It is said that the solution lies within the problem. But when you keep *turning the problem over in your mind* you exhaust your problem-solving abilities and deplete your creative energy.

Once, however, you turn it over to your Higher Power, the pressure is gone. It is no longer your problem, and you can relax, meditate, or rest and quietly go about other activities. Within that leap of faith, that act of turning it over, you have made the space for your Higher Power to act on your problem. Sometimes the answer comes in dreams, sometimes in thoughts that just jump into your consciousness, and sometimes through the words of loving friends.

The answer often comes only when you get out of the way. Try stepping back from your ego and letting go of your analysis. Once you willingly open your heart to the Universal Wisdom we call Higher Power, you will find that you "intuitively know how to handle situations that used to baffle you." (That is one of the promises on page 84 in the Big Book of Alcoholics Anonymous.)

Doing Your Part

A man was standing on his porch during a terrible flood, when a rescue bus came sloshing down the road. The driver yelled to him, "Get on board; we're evacuating the town." "Oh, that's all right," he replied. "I have faith in God. God will save me. Go ahead without me."

The flood waters continued to rise, and he was forced to take refuge in his upstairs bedroom. Soon a rescue worker appeared in a motorboat and called to him, "Quick, hop in! I'll take you to safety!" "No, I'm fine," the man replied. "I have faith in God. He will save me."

The flood waters rose higher. Now the only dry spot left was the very peak of his roof. As the man stood clinging to his chimney, a helicopter flew overhead and threw him a rope ladder. "Quick!" the pilot shouted. "Grab onto the ladder and climb up carefully!" Again the man replied, "No, thanks, I have prayed to God. God will save me. Go help someone else." Unfortunately, the waters continued to rise and the man was drowned.

In time he made it to the pearly gates and found himself standing in front of God. "I'm certainly grateful I was allowed to come to heaven," he said humbly to his Maker, "but one thing I don't understand. I kept praying to you. Why didn't you save me?" "What do you mean?" replied God. "I sent you a bus, a motorboat, and a helicopter! It was *you* who didn't do *your* part."

Simply stated, God helps those who help themselves. So what can you do to tap into that Spirit, that wisdom of Nature, the Higher Power that has kept your body functioning for so many years? For prayer, affirmations, or meditation to work, you must be willing to do your part. You need to cooperate with the Healer within. You must do the things you know deep down inside are right: nurture your body by doing things that sustain and strengthen it, and avoid those things that do damage and are harmful. In other words, you do the footwork, and leave the results up to your Higher Power.

How do you stay in a mode directed always to serve, rather than destroy, yourself. The answer is really so simple we sometimes miss it. Take a step in the direction of faith. You have nothing to lose. Tap into your Higher Power in whatever way works best for you. Affirm that you are cared for and protected by this Force. Turn your will and your life over to the care of a Higher Power as you understand that Higher Power.

Third-Step Prayer

Some of you may want to say a prayer, dedicating your life to your Higher Power, or simply talk to your Higher Power as you would talk to any loving friend. You might want to use a prayer already developed for this exact step. The third step prayer, used by the members of Alcoholics Anonymous, goes like this:

> God, I offer myself to Thee—to build with me and to do with me as Thou wilt. Relieve me of the bondage of self, that I may better do Thy will. Take away my difficulties, that victory over them may bear witness to those I would help, of Thy Power, Thy Love, and Thy Way of life. May I do Thy will always!

Positive Self-Talk: Self-Care

Positive self-talk can emotionally and spiritually support you further. Repeat sayings and affirmations (*affirm*—"to make firm, to make real") until deep in your innermost self you know they are true, and you feel cared for by your Higher Power.

- I cooperate with my Inner Healer by avoiding anything that interferes with my healing, and I actively pursue healthy and healing activities.

- I maintain emotional and mental attitudes that serve me, such as those discussed in Chapter 2.

- By following this program I am developing self-esteem and self-forgiveness.

- It is important not only that I fill myself with nurturing foods and thoughts, but also that I am with people, in places, and around things that nurture me.

- If certain people or places upset me unduly, I find ways to avoid them.

- I am true to myself and my healing.

- I am in the process of breaking old patterns of behavior, so I avoid people who continue to engage in any type of damaging behavior and places where these people are.

- I am beginning to acknowledge my Inner Healer, and I do all the footwork that is my part.

What Are Your Reasons to Go on Living?

Many people never ask themselves their reasons for living and so find their lives without purpose. Those who fail to explore this question may end up wasting their precious days doing things that have no connection with what is really important to them. It is then that a deep, existential loneliness can creep in. "He who has a *why* to live for, can bear with almost any *how*" are the words of Nietzsche from Frankl's *Man's Search for Meaning*. When we go against what we truly value we experience internal turmoil and distress. It "tears us apart," and the distress can lead to many kinds of addictions and other illnesses. One piece of your footwork is to explore your reasons for living.

We live in such a fast-paced world that many of us are so busy "getting there" that by the time we arrive (if we ever do arrive) we may have missed doing what was really important to us. So stop and answer this question: What are my reasons to go on living? If you become emotional when you explore this question, that's okay. Most people do. Go ahead and cry if you need to; that's why we were given tears. We all need to make sure our goals are related to the reasons we want to go on living. Only then will our lives have meaning and purpose.

Setting Goals

Setting goals is necessary to help you develop and maintain a sense of expectancy and accomplishment. In setting goals you are giving your mind and your body messages to live. In setting goals you are investing in your future. When asked the secret to her long and energetic life, Katharine Hepburn replied simply, "Have something you are totally interested in to get up for each and every morning."

Now that you are faced with your own mortality, it is even more important for you to set a clear course for yourself each day. When you set goals, you are affirming your belief in yourself and affirming that you are capable of reaching targets. Setting goals also serves to keep you aware of your responsibility *to* yourself and *for* yourself. *You* are the captain of your ship, and it will go wherever *you* steer it.

All of the people we have talked to who have been living for years with their HIV infection have confirmed to us that goal setting is very important to them. Dan P., diagnosed with AIDS several years ago, thought he was not long for this world. He went out and charged up all of his credit cards to their limits, quit medical school, and moved to Southern California to surf. Several years later he is still trying to pay off his credit cards. He not only lived to get the bills and to surf, he also went back to medical school and graduated. When asked what he would say to those newly diagnosed with HIV infection, he replied, "Tell them not to charge up all their credit cards and to have something for which to live." When Dan's health seemed extremely precarious his goal of becoming a doctor seemed unachievable and therefore irrelevant. So he switched his goal to surfing, a childhood dream that he had long ago discarded, but that once again seemed alluring—and achievable. Dan knew he needed to have a goal, and he displayed a healthy flexibleness in his ability to switch his goal.

Setting goals also helps you stay focused and centered. Going through life without goals is like sailing a ship without a rudder: you may just keep going around in circles. Staying focused on your goals will help you stay on a positive track and give your mind more precise direction. This will enable you to keep out of negative patterns of thinking, self-pity, and fear, which can become self-destructive.

Characteristics of Goals

Goals need to be specific, concrete, measurable, and realistic. They need to answer the questions What, How long, or How much, and When. A goal needs to be measurable so that you will know if you have reached it. For example, "I'm going to listen to my affirmation tape when I'm driving and when I'm around the house doing chores," is better than "I'm going to listen to my affirmation tape more." There is no way to clearly act on or evaluate a nonspecific "more." In Dan's case, his goal was to become a doctor. When he first got AIDS he quit medical school. He has since finished his internship and is applying for a residency.

Keep your goals realistic so you will be able to accomplish them and feel good about yourself. Start off slowly and increase their scope. For example, "I'm going to start by walking ten minutes every morning" is better than "I'm going to run a marathon."

Types of Goals

There are several types of goals we strongly suggest you make for yourself each and every day and write down on a *list*. Make your list the preceding evening or first thing in the morning. This way, as you cross off your list you will feel a sense of accomplishment throughout your day. Keeping a list will help you avoid the feeling of "What have I been doing all day?" or "What do I do next?"

Self-nurturing goals—Do at least one self-nurturing thing a day, whether it be taking twenty minutes to walk through a park, read a book, or take a bubble bath. Do something each day that is pure and simple pleasure for you. You need to, metaphorically, plant your own garden.

Twelve-step goals—Depending upon what step you are currently working, you will need to write down a daily goal for that step. For example, if you are working on step four or eight, you may need to write a list, whereas, if you are on step five or nine you may need to take time to talk with a particular person. You may be only in the reading stage of a step and need a goal such as, I will finish reading the chapter on the third step.

Whole-self healing goals—You need to include all the different aspects of your healing that you are addressing. You may have a doctor's appointment, be going out to get some nutritional supplements, or have a scheduled medication. Include on your list your morning and evening meditation, your affirmations, and your imagery and prayers.

Physical Exercise—It is important to have a goal for your physical exercise. In a study by Dr. George Solomon of long-term survivors of AIDS, exercise was one of the common activities reported. Additionally, at the Center for the Biopsychosocial Study of AIDS at the University of Miami, Dr. Laperriere and others found increases of T4 cells in HIV-positive individuals who engaged in aerobic exercise for 45 minutes three times a week. These increases were comparable to those seen in studies of AZT administration! They also found that aerobic exercise (they used an exercise bike) alleviated anxiety and depression among their HIV-positive subjects.[2]

Whether you are completely well or bedridden, you can still have a daily physical exercise goal. Even in bed you can do leg lifts, arm exercises, or some other type of exercise. Remember, exercise stimulates the production of endorphins, chemicals that decrease pain and instill feelings of well-being. Endorphins bring on the "runner's high," but you don't have to run to feel the benefits!

Social support goals—Social support is always important, and is especially important to your present healing. You need a daily goal that includes making the effort to connect with other people. It may be a twelve-step support group meeting or just calling your sponsor or a friend or a relative.

Remember that not only is your receiving social support very important, but so is your giving support to another. Whether you are totally well, bedridden, or somewhere in between, there is still someone who needs to know that you care and are there for him or her; that is the twelfth step of this program. You do not need to be finished with all the other eleven steps before you start doing the twelfth step. Someone out there needs you. You have much more to give than you may realize. Focusing on another's needs for a while will not only help the other person, but will also help you put things in perspective and feel valuable as a human being. When people in twelve-step programs become absorbed in their own problems they are often encouraged by their sponsors to "Get out of yourself and for God's sake go help someone else!"

Personal "work" goals—By personal "work" goals we mean anything that you do that has meaning to you. It may mean getting promoted or transferred, or it may mean quitting your job and starting a new career. It could refer to helping a sibling, parent, or child, or becoming more socially oriented, or working in some project related to the AIDS crisis.

Many HIV-positive people we have met who have been infected for a long time work with AIDS in general or work specifically with gay, bisexual, hemophiliac, or drug or alcohol groups. There is much work to be done and many ways to do it. In this way you can help others and also give new meaning to your life.

In whatever way you see your life's work, you need to have specific, measurable goals that are in process. For example, if your goal is to paint your bedroom, once your bedroom is painted you need to make a new goal.

Doing It

Take some time now and write down at least one daily goal for each type of goal. Then write one-month, three-month, and six-month goals in each area. As soon as you reach your goals make new ones. If you change your mind about a goal and decide you don't like it or it is not realistic, simply write a new one to replace the one you deleted.

Stay flexible. Often what seems like a good goal may later on look unappealing. Remember, you're taking care of yourself now, so if you need it, give yourself permission to change your mind. It's not a big deal! You really are allowed to change your mind.

Remember to be *true to yourself* and *gentle with yourself*. And although you are writing goals that project into the future, remember to live one day at a time. When you are through writing your goals and doing the footwork, be sure to do a relaxation imagery, such as the one at the end of this chapter.

Action Plans

Each long-term goal (one-month, three-month, or six-month goal) will need an action plan. How exactly are you going to go about reaching your goal? What and who are your resources for such a goal? For example, if you are working on your meditation goal, use a daily meditation book or audiocassette as one of your resources.

Some plans will be very specific and others may be less so, but you definitely need some type of action plan. Use your daily goals to carry out this action plan for a longer range goal. For example, a goal may be to stop drinking alcohol and using mind-altering drugs. The action plan for that goal might be as follows:

1. Checking the phone book for listings of support groups or treatment centers and calling for meeting schedules or information

2. Going to four Alcoholics Anonymous or Narcotics Anonymous meetings a week, or ninety meetings in ninety days (which is recommended if you do not go into a treatment center)

3. Getting a sponsor

4. Avoiding "slippery places," such as bars and nightclubs, and "slippery friends," who use drugs and alcohol.

After getting a sponsor the action plan to remain sober may include suggestions of your sponsor.

Higher Power

Sometimes it is easier to see how faith works in other peoples' lives than in our own. If you know someone who has a working faith in a Higher Power that you admire, it's perfectly okay to borrow his or her faith and Higher Power until you can develop your own. Also, feel free to borrow ours.

Cindy's Higher Power

Today Cindy's Higher Power totally directs her life. She "reports for duty" each morning, trusting that everything that comes up for her that day will ultimately be for her highest good, even though at the time she may not be at all clear about how or why. She mentally pictures herself surrounded and protected by white light and inside a glowing crystal dewdrop suspended by a thin silver thread from her Higher Power.

But it was not always like this. The third step was very hard for her. She is able to do it today only because her concept of God, which she chooses to call her Higher Power, has evolved over time. Her old concept of God was a critical and stern judge who was quick to punish and never gave anyone a break. Cindy had an ovary, fallopian tube, and part of her uterus removed at the age of seventeen and was told she could never have children. At the time she thought that the prognosis was a punishment from God for wanting to have sex. She hadn't actually had sex. In fact, she had lost a boyfriend of three years because she wouldn't have sex with him. "But I thought about doing it. And I had been taught that thinking about a sin was the same thing as committing a sin, so I was in big trouble! It made perfect sense then that God would punish me by taking away my motherhood rights."

"So when I came to the third step I stayed stuck until I realized the reason I could not turn my will and my life over was because I was terrified of what my Higher Power would do with them."

It didn't take Cindy long to notice that all the people who had done the third step had a much more relaxed attitude about life than she did. She wanted the freedom from fear and the childlike spontaneity she saw in these people. "I was always so uptight, waiting for the next shoe to drop."

So "turning it over" was not going to work for Cindy until she transformed her image of her Higher Power. She did that by reading spiritual books, listening to positive, spiritual people, and saying affirmations each morning as she awoke and each night as she went to sleep.

Today she describes her Higher Power this way: "My Higher Power is soft and gentle, loving and kind, forgiving and devoted to my best interest. When I slip into old patterns of behavior that are not coming from my Higher Self, he just picks me up like a lost little lamb whose wool is full of stickers because she went off the open path, and gently pulls the stickers from my wool. As he is holding me, he shakes his head with compassion and says, 'It's okay, I understand. But you'll find that if you stay on the open path more often you'll get fewer stickers and won't get lost as often.' Pure love, pure compassion, pure wisdom, and pure understanding is what my Higher Power is about." Cindy's Higher Power has no gender; Cindy uses the word *he* only out of habit.

Emmett's Higher Power

Emmett's story starts from the other end of the spectrum. By the time he entered the practice of medicine, Emmett was an agnostic. "The main reason I was not an atheist was that it takes great faith to believe that one *knows* there is no God, and it was *belief* itself that was suspect in my mind." Despite this, when he shifted his practice to behavioral medicine and began treating people for psychological problems, a most remarkable thing occurred. He noticed that people got better faster when they had something that they really *believed* in. It seemed that no matter what they were working on—whether it was stopping smoking, losing weight, healing a chronic infection, or developing more loving relationships—having faith in some form of Higher Power seemed to be one of the most powerful factors involved in success.

It didn't matter what their faith was or whether their prayers went to Jesus Christ, the Great Spirit, or the Universal Intelligence. That there was something they believed in deeply seemed to be the key factor. These people had found another source of Power. "I found that people with a deep faith were even able to solve some problems that I continued to have."

Emmett was smoking at that time. He felt badly about his inability to quit. He knew it wasn't good for his health, and because many people came to him for help in kicking their smoking habit, he had to hide his smoking. "I can't tell you how embarrassing it was to look into the eyes of someone who was thanking me warmly for helping him or her kick the same habit that I had been unable to eliminate in my own life."

Soon, however, the truth began to dawn on Emmett. He was beginning to believe in something: the power of faith. Because he had seen it work so often and so well, it became undeniable to him. As his acceptance of a deeper Power within each one of us became stronger, he discovered it within himself. And about his smoking: one of the ways he discovered his Higher Power was through a meditation based on paying attention to his breathing. Each time he breathed in, he filled himself with his Higher Power. He realized that smoking for him was pleasurable because it caused him to take in deep breaths of something that changed his consciousness. With his meditation he can now take in deep breaths of air and feel a change. He stopped smoking and says of his Higher Power, "I now have a very clear sense of my own Higher Power. It is unique and it has evolved to fit my own personal beliefs. If the militant agnostic that I was can do it, I am sure anybody with at least half an open mind can do the same!"

Self-Healing Imagery

As you take in all these ideas and add to your understanding of your Inner Healer, the following relaxation and imagery exercises can help you recognize and delight in your own inner resources. The longer script can be found on page 288.

Part 1: Deep Relaxation

Before you start, eliminate any possibility of interruption or distraction so that you can focus completely upon relaxation, upon peace, and upon your own healing. Unplug the phone, put a sign on the door, let people know that you are going to be taking some time for your own healing and unstressing. Loosen any constricting clothing and sit or lie in a comfortable position.

Part 2: Healing Your Body and Its Immune System

Visualize your immune system. Every cell is dedicated to doing its part for the highest good of the whole. Imagine light flowing toward your cells and surrounding them. Picture your helper cells leading any unwanted cells, bacteria, or viruses to the exit door and giving them a choice. They may either rest or sleep quietly here or else they must leave. Picture your immune cells destroying and ejecting any cells that become hostile. All the cells of your immune system are surrounded by glowing light and are going about their jobs perfectly. Now picture the HIV virus. See the virus as it truly is: weak, sleepy, unwilling and unable to multiply.

Imagine the beam of your consciousness growing smaller and more focused, like a tiny glowing dot suspended in front of your body. Float through the air into that tiny glowing point of pure loving light. Feel yourself being breathed into your body with your next inhalation. You are now traveling through the inside of your own body. Whenever you encounter a dangerous cell, shine a beam of sparkling light on it. Watch as it is wrapped in this light it becomes very drowsy. Your Higher Power flows through you and surrounds it in a soft glow of tranquility and serenity. As this happens all other organs and systems in your body become more peaceful, more harmonious, and more perfectly balanced. Your mind is lucid and serene.

Visualize the air that expands all the little air sacs in your lungs. The oxygen easily flows across a thin membrane and is easily absorbed by the blood. Your skin is clear and of normal color. Moisture and dryness are balanced. Your throat and all the mucous membranes of your body are supple, moist, free, and clear. You have an excellent appetite and can digest all foods well. Your stomach, intestines, and bowel function normally.

Look into the future. Imagine looking at your body in the mirror. It looks healthy and strong. Your weight is normal, you have an excellent appetite, have strong muscles, and are full of energy. Your vision is clear, bright, and well focused. Look at the muscles of your body, the glow of your skin, the sparkle of your eyes, the look of wisdom on your forehead, the look of joy and peace around your mouth. It is clear that the consciousness that inhabits this body listens to this body. This body rests when it is appropriate, exercises when it is appropriate, and takes restful, energizing sleep.

Part 3: Reawakening

Let yourself gradually reawaken, coming back to normal consciousness feeling rested, energized, and healed, or let yourself continue to rest.

Third-Step Affirmations

Turning over your will and your life is something you do consciously and deliberately, maybe even reluctantly, in the beginning. It does not come easily until you've done it enough to experience how well it works. Meanwhile, use these affirmations to help you find those good experiences.

Today I ask only for my will to be in alignment with my Higher Power's will for me.

Today I am in harmony with the inner wisdom of my body.

Today I make firm my healing by the use of affirmations and imagery.

Today I can be honest, open-minded, and willing.

Today I let my Higher Power take care of the outcome while I stay busy doing my part.

Today, as I turn my life over to my Higher Power, the blockages, the difficulties, and the battles disappear, dissolve, or become more manageable.

Today if I feel foggy or unclear, I remember that my Higher Power is clear and that the place where my Higher Power resides deep within me is also clear. I become still and listen for the soft, quiet voice of my Higher Self, my Inner Healer.

Today I am at peace with myself and the world.

FOUR

Awakening Self-Love

STEP FOUR
MADE a SEARCHING and FEARLESS
MORAL INVENTORY of ourselves

MADE *created; caused to exist*

SEARCHING *examining; investigating; close; keen*

FEARLESS *bold, courageous; undaunted*

MORAL *relating to right and wrong*

INVENTORY *a list of items, with their worth
noted; an evaluation*

Step four shows you how to take a good look at your life so that you can better understand and accept yourself. You will then be able to forgive and love yourself, despite activities for which you may feel remorse.

MICHAEL'S STORY

Michael did not want to admit he was gay, let alone admit he had abused drugs and now was HIV positive. When he was told he needed to take a careful look at his life, he was not at all happy. He didn't see what that had to do with anything.

Michael had felt like a failure from a very young age. His

*dad was the high school football coach and having a gay son
would never be okay. Michael tried to be the son his dad
wanted, but somehow always knew he was not. He played
ball both literally and figuratively, denying who he really was
to his family and to himself. He was tormented by constant
self-loathing, acute dissatisfaction, and a loneliness that
reached into the deepest corners of his heart.*

*Michael got involved with drugs and alcohol while he was
in college. That's also when he became sexually active. But
he always brought a token young woman home to family
gatherings. He thought his family must know he was gay on
some level, but he also was sure they did not consciously
acknowledge it. He was so sick of pretending and hated the
old "Have you met anybody you're serious about, dear" routine. When Michael found out he was HIV positive he couldn't
believe it. Stunned and terrified, he stayed drunk and wired
for two months and almost lost his closest friend because of
his hostile attitude.*

*Michael's company ran a random drug screening and told
him he would lose his position if he didn't go in for treatment
for his chemical dependency. He did go for treatment, and it
was there that he was asked to do a fourth-step inventory.
Michael already felt so full of self-hatred and devoid of self-
acceptance that he was sure if he reviewed his past it would
make him feel even more depressed. But, seeing no other way
out of his predicament, he decided to do what was suggested.
He really did want to feel better about himself. Everyone who
had done the fourth step told him it had really made a big
difference in how they felt about themselves and their lives.
Michael sure needed something to help him feel better.*

*He met several guys he really liked at the gay AA and
NA meetings he sought out after he completed treatment.
He envied the joy in their eyes. Michael got a sponsor and
eventually started working on his fourth step in earnest.*

*When he finished, Michael knew he had made the right
decision. He found that he really liked who he was and he
decided to stop pretending to be who he wasn't. He realized
he was not an embarrassment to God and started taking better
care of himself. He went home to tell his mom about both of
his secrets. He figured eventually he would tell his dad, but*

first he wanted his mom to get used to the idea that her son was gay and was infected with HIV.

Not sure exactly how she would react, Michael was simultaneously tense and detached by the time he got the words out. Watching her face cloud with bewilderment and pain, and yet love, concern, and then a new respect, he felt his stomach relax. When he left, after talking a few hours, he knew she would continue coming to terms with his news. He felt lighter, cleansed of years of shame and secrecy.

Michael also found he could look in the mirror and consider loving the guy he saw looking back. Soon that guy would have a talk with his dad. He really understood what his friends had been trying to tell him about the freedom they felt after doing the fourth step. It was only after finding himself that he had gotten the courage to tell his mom. Having gotten rid of that hated secret stuff, he began to notice a small, warm glow of pride within.

Step Four and HIV Infection

Most people suffer some degree of self-alienation owing to incidents in their past. The discomfort that comes with guilt and shame can be very destructive and prevent you from taking care of yourself. Now that HIV infection or AIDS has complicated your life, it is even more vital that you eliminate any energy-draining patterns from your life. Secrets keep you sick.

The fourth step helps you work through secrets and arrive at the other side. Then, unburdened by your past, you can take a deep breath of freedom. You can truly learn to love and accept yourself as you are. You can, while staying in the present, move one day at a time toward healing.

Self-Awareness and Self-Acceptance: The Roots of Self-Love

If your childhood relationship with your parents had been ideal, you would have learned to love and accept yourself fully. But many of us grew up with inadequate positive attention from our parents. Or, perhaps in your parents' attempt to make you understand the rules of life, or in your interpretation of what they said, you missed the message of how very special you are. You may have lost sight of how much potential and magic you have to offer this world. For most of us this is true to one degree or another.

Carl Jung, the famous psychologist, says, "In every adult there lurks a child—an eternal child, something that is always becoming, is never completed, calling for unceasing care, attention and education. That is the part of the human personality that wants to develop and become whole."

The next step in your healing, your becoming whole, is to develop a deep *unconditional love* for yourself. You need to feel for yourself the unconditional love an emotionally healthy parent has for his or her child. Such a love allows you to grow to your fullest potential. So regardless of how little you received in the past, you need to learn to give yourself this love now. Erich Fromm, author of *The Art of Loving,* points out that true love is not an accident, but a conscious choice! To love yourself is a *choice,* a decision that only you can make. It is also a process, an ongoing way of treating yourself, not a once-and-for-all act.

Some people think of self-love as unimportant or even harmful, probably because they often confuse it with false pride. Hence you may have always been encouraged to place other people's needs and desires before your own. In so doing you may have negated your sense of your own worth: your own uniqueness and personal value.

Like the mother who *accepts* her child for who he or she actually is, with his or her strengths *and* shortcomings, you need to accept yourself just as you are, with your strengths *and* shortcomings. Only when you have accepted yourself as you are, "the good and the bad; the beautiful and the ugly," can you capitalize on your strengths. Only then can you overcome or compensate for your weaknesses. You can learn to recognize the difference between *who you were born to be,* and who you *appear* to have become. It is a common mistake to confuse your *self* with your behavior. Especially if you participated in behaviors that did not express your Higher Self, you may have become identified with those behaviors. You may have confused those *behaviors* with who you *are.* It's time to set the record straight.

Positive Self-Talk: Who I Really Am

- I am not my past behaviors.

- Who I am and what I have done are two different things.

- I accept myself as I am, even though I may have parts and behaviors that I am not proud of and choose not to do again.

- I am pure love, hope, and full of possibilities.

- Because I am learning who I really am, my behaviors gradually reflect this truth.

- I love and accept myself just as I am at this moment.

- I am learning how to be happy, joyous, and free.

When Michelangelo was asked how he became inspired to carve the magnificent statue of David, he replied, "When I saw this stone, I saw David. All I did was chip away the stone that was not he." Like Michelangelo, we too must chip away that which is not us.

CASEY'S STORY

Casey was a critical care nurse and loved his work in the emergency room. But owing to an HIV-related illness he became too sick to work. As time went by he felt more and more depressed. Without his job he was no longer "super-nurse" nor could he "save a life a day." He was no longer getting positive strokes or a sense of identity. He felt lost. He didn't have a clue as to who he was anymore. To make matters worse, his roommate said he would move if Casey didn't stop drinking. He was depressed and bitter for a long time, and he resented anyone who tried to cheer him up.

Gradually Casey realized that he had confused what he did with who he was. Eventually he realized that he was not going to die anytime soon and needed to get on with life. More and more restless, he wanted to find an identity beyond what his body could or could not do. But merely surviving was hard work, and there were days when he just wanted to stay in bed and cry. In time, though, he reidentified himself as a special human being. He also became aware again that he was capable of much more than simple behaviors and actions.

With a renewed appreciation of himself, Casey got active in his local NA groups and busy working with a PWA organization. He found he could still "save a life a day" in a way just as meaningful as before.

Affirmations: I Am

Many of our ideas and images of ourselves are unconscious. This includes labels we've given ourselves for making mistakes ("I should never have done that; I guess I'm just a weak-willed person"). Listing all our past behaviors somehow puts them in a new light. When we gain perspective we realize that we are competent, worthy people capable of staying on track, as well as getting off track. Nothing we have done condemns us to repeating behaviors; we can change.

Some changes are easier than others. As you move through your day, these affirmations can help center you in your new sense of wholeness.

- I have my body, but I am not my body.

- I have my feelings and emotions, but I am not my feelings or emotions.

- I have my thoughts and opinions, but I am not my thoughts or opinions.

- I have my actions and behaviors, but I am not my actions or behaviors.

- I have my anger, fear, and sadness, but I am not my anger, fear, or sadness.

- All these are part of me, and yet I am much more.

Guilt

You may feel guilty about or ashamed of some of the things you have done. Remember, each of us is unique and has his or her own special story. Maybe the worst thing *you* ever did was fudge on your income taxes or scream at your children. The point is, no matter *what* it was that you did, if it makes you feel badly about yourself, you need to address it in order to feel better.

The pain of guilt *can* serve a purpose, in the same way that the pain you feel when you sit on a tack serves a purpose. The latter pain tells you that you need to pull out the tack. At this point the pain has served its purpose and is of no further use. Similarly, the pain of guilt ceases to serve any purpose once you recognize that your behavior contradicts your nature. After you identify and begin to change the behavior, you no longer need the guilt.

Guilt can nag at you, causing you to feel helpless, depressed, and angry. It can hold your creativity hostage, and stifle your ability to change. It can make you feel so badly about who you are that you throw in the towel and reject the possibility of change. That feeling quickly can turn into depression, and interfere with your taking care of yourself.

Deep down, you know you are capable of much more. It is this failing to meet *your own standards,* this being untrue to yourself, that makes the guilt weigh so heavily. To move beyond it, it is helpful to acknowledge and accept your guilt. Recognize how it has served you, but let it go. It will be of value the next time you need it. Meanwhile, you are free to redirect your energy toward useful action.

Life Examination and Review

Now that you have a way to deal with the guilt, the fourth step asks you to examine your life. We all need to look back into the past and find meaning in the things that have happened to us and the things that we have done, to take an inventory.

Historically, all great people of religion and psychology have advocated some type of life review, some type of self-reflection. The healing that takes place with self-discovery is awesome. And if you were asked for the most important lessons you have learned, you would quickly see that you learned them through some very painful experiences. Unpleasant as the experience may be, *pain imparts wisdom*. It highlights the truth and emphasizes the value of truth to the body and emotions, *if you are willing to learn*.

This life review may be painful, and it may take some time before you feel willing or ready to do it. That's fine. Remember, these steps are only suggestions. You'll know when and if this suggestion feels right to you. But the lessons gained have made many people feel it was worth it. Once you take a good look at yourself and have some understanding, like Michael, you can start the process of self-forgiveness. And, like Michelangelo, you can chip away that which is not you.

Secrets

There is a saying: "You are only as sick as your secrets." Some things you have done you may never want to remember, let alone examine closely. That's okay. Like most people, Michael felt the same way at first. Some people have done few things they are ashamed of, some have done a lot; most of us fit somewhere in the middle. The truth is that real sickness comes when we have secrets and don't admit them even to ourselves. Once you admit them to yourself, you have the power to accept yourself. This allows self-love, self-forgiveness—and change.

Resentment

The "Big Book" of AA lists resentment as the number one offender. "From it stems all forms of spiritual disease, for we have been not only mentally and physically ill, we have been spritually sick." Resentment is anger, usually based in fear or hurt, that we relive in our minds, often imagining revenge. This reenactment in our minds keeps the initial pain alive and the damage reoccuring. For your own healing, you can benefit from working through your resentments.

One way to do this is to make a list of people, institutions, and principles toward whom you are angry or feel resentment. Think of all the injustices, losses, and outrageously tragic aspects of your HIV infection. List doctors, clinics, rules and regulations, politicians, the FDA, employers, family, acquaintances: everybody and everything with which you are angry.

Next to this listing of people, institutions, and principles, write down how they have negatively affected you. If you have already done a lot of work on your anger, you might still want to just check it out and see if there is more you need to shed. Try writing down twenty-five reasons you are angry with your Higher Power. It's okay to be angry. It's even okay to be angry at your Higher Power. It's not okay to hold a resentment inside, where it can damage you. Let yourself feel the anger! Yell, beat your mattress, wring towels, write letters, and share at meetings or with friends. Get this stuff out before you go on to do your own inventory.

Getting in Touch with Your Wounded Child

As you look back in time, you may also get in touch with the wounded child inside of you. Each of us has a wounded inner child. You may have had parents who did not know how to show love or how to parent. You may have had parents who did a really great job. It doesn't matter. Every person has a wounded child inside—although the degree to which he or she is wounded varies. You need to stop and honor your inner child. Give your inner child your time. He or she deserves it.

Dealing with your wounded inner child can be intense work. If it does not feel like something you want to tackle right now, don't! If you have been severely abused, you probably need to get help with this issue. Steps seven and eight deal more specifically with childhood abuse. We suggest you work with a sponsor, counselor, or a support group.

When you reach your wounded child, it is important to be kind to him or her. In your mind's eye hold that child gently in your arms and rock him or her. Now you have the chance to give to yourself what may have been missing when you were growing up. You have the chance to give yourself a great gift: forgiveness and love.

Some of your anxiety, bitterness, frustration, or depression may be related to the way you were treated in your childhood.

Unfortunately wounded children often grow into people who are abusive. Dr. George Solomon, often referred to as the father of psychoneuroimmunology, did a study in 1988 that supports this point. He found that 6 to 8 percent of the teenagers in the inner city of Newark, New Jersey, were infected with HIV. He wanted to know what factors had led these teenagers to engage in high-risk sexual behaviors and drug abuse. Dr. Solomon found two things: *psychological depression* and a *history of having been sexually molested*. Wounded as children, these teenagers went on to adopt high-risk behaviors that put them in further danger.

Many of us grew up in dysfunctional families: families with alcoholism, drug addiction, or physical, mental, emotional, spiritual, or sexual abuse. If we don't deal with these issues, we unconsciously allow the abusers to continue abusing us in our later lives. That is, we continue reacting in dysfunctional ways as a result of our original abuse. Keep in mind that most abuse was unintentional, and this is not to blame anyone. But to ignore that it happened perpetuates the power it holds over your adult life.

Even if you do not react with any of the behaviors that were found in the teenagers in Newark, if you were abused, your self-esteem was damaged. You no doubt have difficulty in relationships, especially with trust and abandonment issues. You may end up sabotaging any relationships that may be healthy, or unconsciously choosing unhealthy ones. Additionally, you may often feel deep anger or sorrow or have difficulty with depression or unexplainable generalized anxiety.

Abuse comes in many forms. You did not have to be beaten, and your parents did not have to be alcoholics, to have affected you in some adverse way. Many children are damaged by the absence of a workaholic parent, even though that parent may give his or her children many material possessions in an attempt to make up for the lack of love and attention.

You are *not* to blame for any childhood abuse! Again, remember dysfunctional parents of all sorts, instead of improving their inability to parent, often blame their children. It is really important that you understand this. The legal age for driving is sixteen for a reason other than length of legs. Legally, anyone under that age is not considered aware enough to make serious choices. You could not choose with full clarity a lot of things for which you may have been blamed. And, sad to say, many of us accepted the blame and

118

ended up apologizing to the people who abused us for "making them" abuse us! You can surely cry for that child now. You can even get angry. If this was true for you, throw some pillows and beat your mattress. Express your disgust for such a sick and sad situation.

Another useful tool is to make a list of all the people who have harmed you. Even if you do not feel the harm fits into the category of abuse, list anyone who harmed you in any way. As you are writing, you may feel like describing what happened or writing a letter (which you need not send) to the person or persons who harmed you. If you do, go ahead.

Let yourself feel your anger and grief. You may spend a fair amount of time crying here. That's okay. These tears are probably *very* old, and you deserve to shed them. Even reading about this may have moved you. If it did, let it out. Let yourself heal those old, deep wounds.

Writing a letter to your inner child is also very helpful. You can let that child know that you understand and will be there to support him or her from here on. Let your inner child know that you are in charge now and there are new rules. Today you can make a decision to take care of your inner child. You may even want to get involved with "inner-child groups," which deal specifically with these issues. Several excellent books on this subject are listed in the resource section of the appendix.

Pride and Fear

Often the basic human instincts and innate drives that have served for millennia to keep the human race alive—such as the desire to be assertive and to realize one's dreams, or to care for and nurture another—are also those that end up tyrannizing us. Most of our misdeeds have been the result of an inappropriate use of these basically desirable instincts, which are necessary for life. Many psychologists believe that pride and fear often influence other instincts and cause them to go awry. It is useful to spend some time looking honestly, openly, and willingly at the role of pride and fear in your life.

There is a kind of pride that is healthy and basic to life. This kind of pride is the opposite of shame. We can see it in the joyful smile of the baby who stands in his crib for the first time or the child who finally succeeds in tying her shoes.

But pride is dangerous when you identify your ego too much with actions or objects. Then, instead of honoring and caring for what you *are,* you begin to defend what you have *done* or what you *own.*

This kind of pride may lead you to rationalize and justify, and place unreasonable demands on yourself and others. Your pride may step in to justify your responding excessively, and fear may keep you from seeing what you are doing. This is the kind of pride that "goeth before a fall." Pride is a virtue, but too little or too much endangers all of us.

Fear is essential to survival. Each e-motion is a survival mechanism to put us "in motion." Fear protects us by warning us when something potentially harmful may happen. But when fear is too great or when it is misdirected, it itself can be deadly. It then becomes the source of further unreasonable thoughts and acts. Your fears may, for instance, have driven you to become angry when your needs were not met or envious when others were recognized while you were not.

Everyone starts with good intentions, but our spirits may become distorted even while in the womb. Just as it is with good seeds that do not find fertile soil, these intentions may not have been nurtured, and instead, harmful thoughts, feelings, and actions may have been rewarded. Recognizing the fundamental goodness of your intentions is essential, now that you have the power to nurture them.

Positive Self-Talk: Accepting Good Intentions

- I was always doing the best I could, even though I may have been doing it out of confusion, shame, or fear.

- I am learning to love my hurt inner child.

- At my core I am a loving person.

- This step will help me forgive my wounded inner child and show my child new and better ways of acting.

- At my center is peace.

- My heart and mind are becoming more honest, open, and willing.

Dropping the Guilt and Shame

Please be careful not to use this fourth step as an exercise in self-abuse. If you feel you are to blame for your or someone else's HIV infection or risk of infection, you need to spend more time with your sponsor or counselor working through this. Most people became infected before they even knew how the infection was transmitted. A few people were exposed hundreds of times and did not become infected, and others were infected after one exposure. One baby from a set of twins can be born infected and the other not be infected. This is an inadequately understood disease.

Even if you became infected owing to some behavior that you were fully aware was highly risky, keep in mind that many of these behaviors are part of the disease of addiction—such as drug and alcohol abuse and compulsive sex. Any addictive process has denial built into it. That's what makes it an addiction! If addictive diseases were not so hard to manage, there would be no need for Alcoholics Anonymous or any other twelve-step programs, so please be gentle with yourself.

Many people know when their acts are of a life-threatening nature. If they could just stop, there would be no smokers, no overweight people. Alcoholics would quit after the first bad hang-over, drug addicts would stop when they ran out of money, and abused women would leave after the first slap. Denial—unconsciously pretending what is true is not true—is the nature of addictive diseases and is very difficult to change. Knowledge is often not enough; *denial keeps it from being enough.* So to feel shame and to blame ourselves is not helpful and is potentially harmful. When we feel "less than," owing to our shame and self-blame, we are reluctant to honestly look at ourselves, afraid we will find more things about which to feel "less than." In this way shame and self-blame keep us blind to the things we need to discover as we remain hostile toward, and unconsciously dishonest with, ourselves. Shame and self-blame can hold us prisoner in the prison of "less-than" if we are not careful.

The way to make the most out of this fourth-step inventory is to be totally honest and totally self-responsible: "Yes, this is what happened. Yes, this is my pattern. Yes, I assume responsibility for my part, which gives me the power to change it." But remember, *responsibility* is not the same as *blame*. If you use this step to further wallow in shame or self-blame, you are only causing more damage and will hurt your chances for change. This does not mean that you shouldn't feel sad or emotional. But feeling sad is different from narcissistically whipping yourself. Please be careful here; it is a very fine line.

Your Inventory

As you will probably discover from doing an inventory, most mistakes are the same ones, repeated again and again. The faces and places may change, but the actions and feelings usually fit the same basic script.

Like most of us, you probably didn't always know how to express your true intentions in responsible action. What you thought you were doing, or what you meant to do or say, may not have worked out the way you intended. This inventory, and truly knowing yourself, can be a concrete step in becoming true to your intentions and yourself. Steps six and seven will complete this process.

It is easiest to start your inventory by asking yourself some questions. Be sure to be rigorously honest. The only one you can fool by not being honest is yourself. You may have used rationalizations as excuses for crazy and damaging conduct. You would not have needed rationalizations unless you were going against your basic nature, unless you were being unfaithful to yourself. Honor this realization and its source.

Try dropping the word *blame* from your vocabulary and the action of blaming from your life. Instead look at those things you really have control over: your behavior and your responses. Try holding yourself *accountable* without berating yourself with *blame*.

To give your mind direction, it is helpful to work in chrono-logical order as you take inventory of your life. Five-year increments are a good way to start. When a person's name pops into your mind, write it down. You can use these names later on for further self-forgiveness steps. Be thorough and honest. Hide nothing. You want a full, "no dirt under the rug" kind of housecleaning.

The following questions are intended to serve merely as a guide. Some of them may not apply to you, but really think about each one before you decide. Most of them apply to all of us to some degree. Keep yourself honest, open-minded, and willing. You'll probably think of many other questions not on this list, and you'll want to include them. While doing this review, whenever you remember anything, it indicates that the event made a mark on your consciousness, so write down what happened.

So far in this program this process may be the one that you most want to skip. But if you really want to get the most out of the twelve-step philsophy, we encourage you to consider doing an inventory. To be alive and healthy, we all need to work at every level: physical, emotional, mental, and spiritual. Whatever you may have done belongs in this inventory. No matter how you feel about certain acts, they are perfectly acceptable as historical facts; you have already lived through them all. Admitting them helps free you from repeating them, so give yourself credit for every item in your inventory. The harder it is to write down, the more important is the lesson it holds for you.

Positive Self-Talk: Willingness to Look

Before, during, and after you begin your look at your life, use these sayings to affirm the positive spirit of this venture:

- A life of self-hatred and self-denial is no life. I want a life.

- I've made a decision to live life to the fullest, and to do that I need to learn to forgive myself.

- I see my past behavior as that of a misdirected soul trying to avoid pain and searching for love.

- My Higher Power has forgiven me a long time ago. Now it's time for me to forgive myself.

- I am learning to love and accept myself despite my flaws. In this way I can have enough self-esteem to change.

- I make a decision to do this life review.

- I will learn from my patterns and change what I need to change.

Sexuality

Most of us wish that in some ways we had handled our sexuality differently. Let's look at sexual behavior first.

We're not making any judgments about sexual orientation or numbers of partners, and neither should you. But whether you are gay or straight, you need to look at past sexual behaviors, whether it was knowingly having unsafe sex or being an insensitive lover, anything that you feel uncomfortable about in any way. If you come from a dysfunctional family, especially one in which drugs or alcohol were abused, you were not taught appropriate ways of handling life or managing stress. You may have used sex as one way of dulling your emotions.

People abuse themselves and others sexually for many reasons. Out of fear of intimacy and as a reaction to their own sexual or physical abuse, people may become sexually unresponsive, promiscuous, or overweight. Others use their sexuality as a means of manipulation, and can end up feeling like their entire worth depends on their ability to sexually entice. We do not want you to beat yourself up over this. You only need to be honest with yourself and take a good look at your patterns. Study after study indicate that abused children become adults who abuse themselves and others. This program is a way to stop that!

We know it is tough, but it is really helpful to look at these matters. You may feel like crying as you read these questions. That's okay; go ahead and cry. Tears are healing. It's tough accepting responsibility for yourself. And it's essential.

QUESTIONS: How, when, and with whom did my sexual self-indulgences damage me or others? Who was hurt and how badly? Did I damage my partner or my spouse in any way? Did I spoil a marriage or relationship? Did I, in any way, injure my children? Did I jeopardize my or someone else's self-respect or reputation?

How did I act when frustrated in sexual matters? Did I become vengeful or depressed? Did I take it out on other people? Did I use rejection or self-pity as an excuse for promiscuity? Did I endanger myself or another by certain sexual acts? Did I justify or blame others for my behavior? Did I need love, but settle for sex? Did I use sex like some people use drugs: to escape dealing with reality, or to avoid psychic pain? If I did, I not only dishonored and disrespected my partners, but, equally important, I dishonored and disrespected myself.

Balance

True humility can result only from an honest appraisal of all your thoughts, words, and deeds. To have true humility you need to look at the other side of the coin. Be honest here too. To accept this part of the truth is to nurture yourself and to honor a beautiful part of you.

QUESTIONS: In what ways was I a good partner? How was I kind and considerate? When was I warm and loving? In what ways was I a caring partner, a selfless parent? When did I go out of my way to be understanding to my partner? How did I try to spare another unnecessary pain? In what ways did I try to help the people close to me feel good about themselves? What did I do to protect myself and my sexual partners?

Money and Job

Fear, greed, possessiveness, and pride often play into how we pursue financial security. Honest answers here open the door to new options.

QUESTIONS: What part did I play in my own financial instability or insecurity? Did fear and a sense of inferiority about my abilities destroy my confidence? Did I cover up my feeling of inadequacy by cheating, lying, bluffing, or evading responsibility? Did I complain and gripe that no one recognized my talents, or overcompensate and play the big shot? Did I steal, work quick deals, gamble, "borrow" money with no intention of paying it back, or fail to support myself or my family properly? In a fit of self-justification did I walk out on a job or badmouth my fellow employees or boss? If the actions of others were the cause of my conflict, what measures did I take to adjust myself to the situation? If it was a completely unacceptable situation, why did I stay? Did I enjoy having something about which to complain? Did I revel in the victim stance or love feeling self-righteous?

Balance

Many times you may have contributed more; been a positive influence. Look now at those times. This is the concrete for your new foundation.

QUESTIONS: In what ways did I act responsibly in my financial affairs? In what ways did I provide well for my family? How was I a good employee? In what ways did I treat my co-workers as I would like to be treated? In what ways did I go out of my way to do the right thing, when the wrong thing would have been easier? When was I honest when I could have gotten away with being dishonest? How did I handle money responsibly? In what ways did I contribute to a good workplace environment?

Relationships

The most common symptoms of emotional insecurity are self-pity, anger, worry, and depression. It is important to look at all of your personal relationships that have a recurring theme of discomfort. Find out what you were doing to keep this merry-go-round turning, so that *you* can stop it and get off—and onto a new and different ride that offers you a fresh and more satisfying way of relating to people.

Be easy on yourself here. Relationships are probably the most difficult area for everybody. They seem to bring out the best and the worst in all of us. If you come from a dysfunctional home, you certainly did not have good role models for relationships. We can only do as well as we have been taught. And unless you uncover your past, you can't discard what doesn't work.

QUESTIONS: What relationships, present and past, caused me anxiety, bitterness, frustration, or depression? In what ways was I at fault? Did I choose poorly? Did I stay in an abusive relationship too long? Did I play martyr, in an "after all I've done" role? Did I dominate people or depend on them too much? Were my demands all-encompassing demands? Did I become more insecure and manipulating through games that eventually drove people away from me? Did I then feel hurt, persecuted, and vengeful? Did I suffer because of my own need to control others? Was I always either struggling to be in charge or whining because I allowed myself to be dominated?

Balance

To be fair with yourself, take inventory of all the positive things you brought to your relationships. A lot of you is healthy and good. You need to realize and accept that part too. Honor and call upon it.

QUESTIONS: In what ways was I selfless? In what ways did I try to make things right? When did I apologize for my part in arguments? When was I the first one to stop a fight and talk things over in an adult way? How was I a good parent, child, sister, brother, friend, lover? When did I feel like doing or saying something that would hurt the other person but stopped myself? When did I control my temper? When did I go out of my way to try to understand the other person's point of view? When did I approach situations and people with a loving and giving attitude? When did I forgo playing the victim or the persecutor?

Take some time and think of areas of your life that were not covered by these questions. You may as well include them while you're at it. Our questions are not a complete list.

Facing the Truth

After you've completed your inventory you will have a long list of situations in which you can clearly see how you have helped to create your own misery. You can also see where you created your own success by acting lovingly and responsibly. Probably everything you need to forgive yourself for was just your way of trying to be happy. That's all any of us ever really wants: just to feel good inside. Somehow we just couldn't get it, or if we got it we couldn't keep it for very long or were afraid of losing it.

This is not an effort to justify behavior; it is just how we human beings are. Because you may not have had very good tools for handling life's stressors, you may have chosen to run from them. You may have used other people, sex, work, drugs, or alcohol to escape feeling bad.

You can no longer escape. Look where it got you. Life is here and you are learning how to face it. HIV infection has probably really made that soberingly clear. Now you can clearly see what about your life needs to be different so you can move toward wholeness, toward healing all of yourself.

It's important to forgive yourself and others and go on from here. The only way you can forgive yourself is to take full responsibility for *your* actions. The upcoming steps cover this further. You are seeking to understand *your* behavior, which differs from blaming other people for what you did. *You* did these things. They are *your* responsibility. Finding out how your inner yearnings became misdirected acts is liberating and strengthening.

Balance in Your Life

In your review you may have noticed that your body took quite a bit of abuse if you "looked for love in all the wrong places." Between anxiety, overindulgence in sex, drugs, alcohol, tobacco, misuse of food, and deprivation of sleep, it is actually amazing that the human body can do so well for so long. Another revelation!

It's also amazing how people who have engaged in the least abuse sometimes carry the greatest remorse. Maybe you never smoked, did drugs or alcohol, or abused your body. Many people who are infected did not! Nancy became infected from a lover before she started using safe sex. She lived in an ashram and had never used alcohol or drugs. But she realized that there were still some changes she needed to make. Most people do need to make some changes regarding worrying, control, ambition, miscommunication, resentments or other issues.

We all really need more balance in our lives. You can't just look at the things about you that you want to eliminate. Look at the bright side of yourself again, the side that needs further development. You have a lot of wonderful qualities. You have done many wonderful things. Review the following list and write down in what ways you demonstrate these and any other qualities that you like in yourself.

QUESTIONS: Am I humble, accepting both my strengths and my weaknesses? Do I admit my mistakes? Am I able to be myself, without pretense? Am I generous and willing to share? Am I patient with myself and others? Am I able to feel good about my accomplishments and others' accomplishments? Am I forgiving? Do I try to be honest? Do I accept others as they are, allowing for imperfections? Am I grateful for the people and things in my life? Do I avoid comparing myself with others? Am I sympathetic toward others and toward myself? In what ways do I use my wonderful mind and body to better a tiny piece of this world? What are my special talents: creating, cooking, talking with people, working with my hands, writing, dancing, singing, designing, running, laughing?

Spend time reflecting on these questions. Pretend you are writing a letter of recommendation for yourself. Pull away from yourself. Really look at all the many things that are so special about you and write them down: "I recommend this person for the following reasons." "These are this person's special qualities." "And these are the reasons this person is a good friend."

We all tend to be our own harshest critics and worst enemies. Switch this to being your best friend. Do for yourself what you would do for your best friend. If becoming a fully mature adult is about being our own best friends, we need to start lightening up on ourselves.

Think back to some of your most treasured accomplishments. It might have been earning an Eagle Scout badge, playing a piano piece, working in your garden, earning a big check, moving into a new office, or watching the light in the eyes of a loved friend happy to see you. Bathe yourself in these positive feelings and memories for a while.

Dealing with Your Feelings

It may take you days or even weeks to complete your life review. Every time you are done working on it, it's important to do a relaxation exercise. *This is a deep and emotional process.* You may experience many different feelings, from grief to anger to newfound satisfaction. If you are working with a counselor, share these feelings with him or her. Talking will help. You will be sharing what you write when you get to step five, but you may want to share your strong feelings as you go along.

Some feelings toward other people may develop or reemerge as you take inventory of your life. When they do, just start writing exactly what you would like to say to that person. Some of it may hurt. Some of it may be very angry. That's okay. Life isn't fair. You may have been dealt some low blows. This is where you beat the mattress again, and maybe scream into a pillow. You will need to do a relaxation process to recenter yourself every time you're done working on this process.

Imagery for Letting Go

The following experience provides a way for the deeper levels of your mind to release behaviors, feelings, people, thoughts, and beliefs that no longer serve to enrich your life. Many cultures provide specific rituals for times of passage, letting go of one phase of life and moving into another. The deeper levels of the mind are then much better able to move into the new phase. The following imagery can serve as your own personal ritual. Its design is partly based on time-tested rituals from many cultures. The full script is on page 292.

Part 1: Deep Relaxation

Before you start, eliminate any possibility of interruption or distraction so that you can focus completely upon relaxation, upon peace, and upon your own healing. Unplug the phone, put a sign on the door, let people know that you are going to be taking some time for your own healing and unstressing. Loosen any constricting clothing and sit or lie in a comfortable position.

Part 2: Letting Go

Gradually you are lifting up and floating through space and time. As you enjoy this floating feeling, imagine a container in front of you, a container in which you will be able to place all those things it is time for you to let go.

Float back through time to collect those things from your recent or distant past that you wish to let go. You and your box are surrounded by the glow of loving light.

If you are at the stage of letting go of negative ways of thinking, when a negative way of thinking occurs to you, hold it in your mind for a moment, and as you breathe out, let it flow into your box. Let it go.

If you are at the stage of letting go of inappropriate habits or behaviors, visualize one briefly and with your next breath out, breathe it into that special box. Let go.

If you are at the stage of letting go of outmoded ways of being, see one briefly in your mind's eye, and then let it flow out into the container.

If you are at the stage of letting go of certain people, visualize a person in your mind, and then breathe him or her out into the container.

Imagine closing the lid and fastening it securely. Stand in front of your container and meditate for a few moments. Say goodbye to the container and all its contents.

Surround it with white light, and picture your container beginning to float away from you. As it becomes more distant it looks smaller and smaller. In the distance you can see the pure white light radiating from it. Feel the warmth of that light as it reaches you and flows over you.

Focus now on the center of your being, and see it as a seed sending roots into the ground and leaves into the air. And any time any concerns or worries come along, you can breathe them into your container.

Part 3: Reawakening

Gently feel yourself returning, coming back full of enthusiasm and hope. Or you can choose to drift off into a deep, relaxing sleep.

Fourth-Step Affirmations

To maximize your health and serenity, you need all the energy you can get. Making peace with your past through this inventory frees tremendous resources within you, which then help you create exactly the life you want. Use these affirmations to help yourself do this.

- Today my past serves to help me find out who I really am.

- Today I choose to be responsible for my thoughts, words, and deeds.

- Today I am learning to love myself better.

- Today I am learning to understand myself more.

- Today I know my past behaviors are not who I am.

- Today I know that I am a worthwhile person.

- Today I choose to release guilt and shame.

- Today I choose to forgive myself.

FIVE

Sharing

STEP FIVE

**ADMITTED to the God of our UNDERSTANDING
to ourselves, and to another human being
the EXACT NATURE of our WRONGS**

ADMITTED *acknowledged; confessed*

UNDERSTANDING *knowing; comprehending;
apprehending the meaning*

EXACT *accurate; precise; closely correct*

NATURE *quality; sort*

WRONGS *not what ought to be; what is not right;
unjust acts*

Step five can release you from the burden of guilt for any real or imagined mistakes you have made. This release becomes possible when you share your story with another person. With this act of sharing you are essentially embracing the entire step, because in admitting your faults to another person you are admitting them to yourself and your Higher Power. You already know your secrets, but may attempt to minimize, justify, or deny them so that their true importance or reality is denied. To humble ourselves enough to admit our wrongs—to ourselves and to our Higher Power—can be a very cleansing and nurturing act. Such honesty can be said to heal the soul. Sharing with another human being, although terribly

133

frightening at first, has been the key to much serenity and peace for millions of people.

Step Five and HIV Infection

The courageous work suggested in step four now becomes even more heroic in the sharing of that inventory. Society is becoming better informed, but most infected people still feel alienated and ashamed. If you were already in any minority group before your infection, the loneliness of that status may now be compounded. In sharing the fifth step you can abandon the lonely shadow that may seem to follow you. You can reconnect with and rejoin the human race. This is no time for the added stress of unshared secrets. Only after you have done the fifth step can you realize what a joy it is to "drop the rock," and move closer to healing.

WILLIAM'S STORY

William was a member of AA. He had been sober for more than two years, yet he had not written out his fourth-step inventory or shared it with anyone. He hesitated and was miserable because his secret was "too horrible" to tell anyone.

William was raised a Mormon on a farm in Iowa. His family was very religious and had rigid expectations. As a teenager he had had sex with his sister. How could he ever admit that? No one would understand. He kept putting off doing his life review, citing a million reasons for not having time to get to it. His insides writhed in shame, fear, and dread.

He stayed miserable for more than two years, sober but in hiding from himself and his secret. When the emotional pain finally became so excruciating that he thought he might start to drink again, he took a huge, healthy risk. With his throat tight from anxiety, he spoke about his past with his AA sponsor. This person had never had sex with his sister, but said he knew of other people who had.

The relief that William felt was miraculous. His listener obviously accepted what he had revealed without rejecting or damning him. Without condoning William's acts, this man's voice conveyed compassion and concern. William swallowed. This time his throat was tight from tears and sadness welling up in great, wracking waves. Because he had let go, he was finally able to purge himself of his terrible guilt.

Honest, Open Sharing

"No man is wise enough by himself," is an ancient proverb. One way to gain true insight is to allow another human being to look at who you are. You may be too wrapped up in it all and therefore lack a clear perspective. Having had the courage and determination to review your life, your behaviors and reactions, the patterns that have been so much a part of you, the fifth step invites you to share this with another human being. The actual writing of the life review was partially cleansing, but now you can actually give it away: *let go of it all.*

The wisdom of the ages shows that all wise men and women, be they rulers or paupers, seek counsel from spiritual advisers, those who can give them objective opinions. This release, this sharing, can be quite beneficial. Whether it be in the confessional, on a therapist's couch, over a cup of coffee, or in a foxhole, the process of sharing who we are, and where we have been, heals us and helps us grow. It allows us a new perspective on who we are, what we do, and why we do what we do. Self-disclosure to a trusted person moves us toward wholeness.

In the act of sharing yourself with someone else, you can become more accepting of the parts of yourself that you have denied or kept hidden. This admittance of your entire being, and acknowledgment of both the pretty and the ugly, becomes an inner completion. You need no longer hide or yearn for the fulfillment of the seemingly vast hole inside your gut, for you now have the tools to give importance to your *entire* self, in the presence of someone else, yourself, and your Higher Power.

Sharing with others takes the dark, musty secrets out of the closet. It allows the light and fresh air of the new day to reveal to you the truths that need to be looked at, truths that can enable you to change the things you need to change while accepting all that you are.

Other Disclosure Issues

Separate from the sharing of the fourth-step inventory, you may have other issues regarding with whom you should share intimate details of your life. If you are gay you may be totally open or you may be totally in the closet. We feel a middle-of-the-road approach is probably the best one if you are presently holding this secret or any other secrets, such as HIV infection or addiction.

Those who are gay tell us that the more people that know and accept this aspect of themselves, the better they feel—up to a point, that is. It is best to start off with someone you think will hold no prejudice. Most find that to be a brother, mother, close friend, or counselor. Be careful to avoid telling anyone who could place your job, home, or life in jeopardy. It's awful but true that homophobia is rampant, and especially if you are new to disclosure you need to protect yourself. It is important for any type of disclosure that you choose safe people so that you start out with some successes and feel good about them. Everyone who needs that information for your well-being should be told, such as your doctor and your counselor. Gradually, as you break out of isolation and start accepting who you are, you will become more comfortable.

The same suggestions apply to your HIV status and any addiction. If telling a person will make you feel better, is important to your well-being, and will not initiate prejudice that could harm you in any way, then go ahead. But to proclaim your HIV or addiction status just for shock value will cause you untold grief. You may be unconsciously looking for rejection to validate your lack of self-acceptance, and this is certainly one way to get it. But you may not only feel rejection, but, depending on where you live, also lose a job or home.

Some very brave people, such as Betty Ford and those in the group ACT-UP, choose to make a statement for these causes. They recognize their public statements as their choice, feel strongly about their purpose, and are fully aware of the possible ramifications of their speaking out. Thank God for these people; someday you may be one of them. Remember that it requires incredible courage.

Your personal truth is your own, and you have the right to pick and choose with whom you share it—not out of shame, but out of respect for yourself. Most people still do not understand homosexuality, HIV infection, or addictions, and may respond with fear, anger, or prejudice. Recovering alcoholics have known this for years. In the beginning they are careful with whom they share their stories, but after a while it's no longer an issue and they tell whomever they choose, whenever they choose to do so. Because of this openness some people may feel it is okay to bring up their sexuality or HIV status in an AA meeting. Unfortunately, in some meetings you will receive support and in others you may not. Ask people what meetings and what people are safe. There are gay meetings and there are meetings especially for HIV-positive people. It's a shame not all meetings and not all people are safe, but that is still the case. Recovering people are still people and some hold strong prejudices. The wise person gets out of the closet but picks confidantes carefully until he or she has a circle of close, supportive friends who know his or her secret. Then it is easier for that person to start telling others.

Connection with Another

Feeling your best starts with feeling connected, feeling a part of the human race. Handling any type of disclosure carefully assures you a greater chance of feeling that connection. Seeing those things that make you similar to others means discovering that you are not so "different," not so "bad." It is comforting to know that other people have felt the same feelings you have, done the same things you have done, and suffered as you have suffered. Once you can identify yourself as a special person, unique and yet similar to others, it's easier to receive as well as give comfort and support. Sharing your life story has powerful benefits.

For this experience of sharing your fourth-step inventory to be rewarding and fulfilling, it is important that you tell your story to the right kind of person. You need someone who will not be personally injured or affected by the content of your story. Therefore it is not appropriate for you to tell your story to someone with whom you have an intimate relationship, such as a spouse, partner, or parent. Some of your unpleasant behavior may cause the other person pain if he or she becomes aware of it, and you cannot make a clean sweep of things at the expense of another. Also, you are less likely to say what you *need* to say.

You may choose a minister or priest, your sponsor, a counselor or therapist, a nurse, a doctor, a volunteer, or a good friend. You may know the person, or someone may recommend an understanding stranger. Sometimes a stranger, so long as he or she understands your purpose, can be the perfect person to help you with the insight you need. You could ask around and find a compassionate person who fits the bill. You could call a Catholic church and find out when confessions (now called reconciliations) are held, and anonymously talk to a priest. Check beforehand, though, to make sure the priest understands twelve-step programs and knows what a fifth step is. Not all do, but many recovering priests are familiar with twelve-step programs. Indeed, for those who are interested, there are even quite a few recovering alcoholic gay priests who would be happy to help you. Ask around at AA/NA meetings for a referral to such a person.

Release and Insight, Not Criticism or Punishment

Explain to whomever you choose to tell your story that you are not asking for penance or punishment. You might even have that person read the fourth and fifth chapters of this book. You are not asking for a scourging or a lecture. Nor will you *accept* a scourging or a lecture! Sharing is for release and insight. Explain that this process is part of a mental, emotional, and spiritual purging that clears the way to wholeness. Let the person know that you welcome any insights he or she may have, and that you are trying to identify patterns in order to facilitate clarification, acceptance, and change. The whole point of this is to uncover, discover, and discard any behaviors that do not serve you or others.

Twelve-Step Programs as Resources

Another excellent source of people who understand this fifth step is Alcoholics Anonymous, Narcotics Anonymous, Adult Children of Alcoholics, Al-Anon, or any other twelve-step programs. The steps are the same in any twelve-step program; only the emphasis differs. Look for a twelve-step group member whom you trust; he or she should have completed this same step and fully understand its purpose.

If you are homosexual, you can find out about gay AA meetings by calling your local AA. Or you could attend an open meeting (open meetings allow people who are not alcoholics to attend) and ask the secretary for the name of someone with whom you could share your fifth step. You may meet someone at the meeting with whom you feel a kinship; if he or she has done this step and understands your intentions, this may be a good person to choose to listen to your life review.

Most members of any of the twelve-step programs have felt deep and bitter remorse for activities they engaged in while using their drug of choice (alcohol, food, drugs, sex, gambling, and so on). They can relate to the feelings of guilt, of not being okay, of being "less than," and of alienation: feelings we all experience when we are not meeting our own standards. Most members of these groups felt emotionally torn apart for a long time before joining the group. You need, however, to be certain to pick someone who has no prejudice toward you if you are a member of *any* minority group. It would be helpful to check that out first.

Doing It

You may want to make a list of at least three people or three ways you can find a person with whom you can share your fourth step inventory. Making a schedule and arrangements to share your story with these people may keep you from procrastinating. Before you read your inventory, write down the names that are on it on a separate sheet of paper. You will use them in step eight.

As you venture into this extremely important step, you may feel some fear and anxiety before your meeting with another person. Sometimes old guilt and anger toward yourself may emerge despite your best intentions, even after you have confided in the other person. Here again, the relaxation process is very valuable. You want to relax with the Loving Light Imagery from step one or the Spiritual Attunement Imagery from step two before and after your meeting to keep your stress level at a minimum. Stay relaxed and trust your Higher Power.

After you have done your fifth step, you may want to burn the inventory. As you watch it go up in smoke, rejoice in your rebirth. Out of the ashes you can begin anew. Repeat the following affirmations whenever you are considering using the philosophy of the fifth step or actually doing the fifth step. Most of us need to encourage ourselves to take this step.

Positive Self-Talk: Opening Up

- Telling my story, letting go of all that personal history, will be a wonderful catharsis.

- I release those secrets that have kept me apart from others, kept me feeling different, isolated.

- I will open up and share.

- I will feel reconnected and free!

Fifth-Step Affirmations

Today I can trust this process.

Today I can confide in someone.

Today I can cry tears of happiness and relief as I feel the weight of my life lifted from me.

Today I know that although this may be one of the most difficult things I have ever done, I can do it.

Today I know that this process is for my growth and peace of mind.

Today I feel connected to my sisters and my brothers, a part of the bigger whole.

Today feelings of alienation are replaced by feelings of belonging and compassion.

Today I am free to let go of the past. I feel clean and new.

Today I am at peace with myself and the world.

SIX

Surrendering

STEP SIX

BECAME ENTIRELY READY to have
the God of our UNDERSTANDING REMOVE
all of these DEFECTS of CHARACTER

BECAME *passed from one state to another;
grew; changed*

ENTIRELY *wholly; completely; fully; altogether*

READY *fit for immediate use; offering itself at
once; willing*

UNDERSTANDING *knowing; comprehending;
apprehending the meaning*

REMOVE *to take away; to cause to leave*

DEFECTS *faults; absence of something necessary
or useful to perfection*

CHARACTER *the peculiar qualities impressed by
nature or habit on a person, which distinguish
him or her from others*

Step six begins the restoration of your peace of mind about
yourself and any behaviors that you wish to change. The
alternative—to reject change—can be devastating, as Andrew's
story shows.

ANDREW'S STORY

Andrew hated his father, who had repeatedly humiliated him and his mother. Andrew was glad when he was old enough to move out of the house. He thought it would end there. Instead, he found himself drawn to other men who were abusive to him. He developed physical ailments and was angry and depressed at the same time. He finally went to a health clinic and found out he had AIDS. Paralyzed with fear, he refused to let his parents know.

Several of Andrew's friends pointed out how his hatred for his father was hurting him. He had heard all that "airy fairy love and forgiveness bullshit" from people in support groups and was not impressed. He was unwilling to even consider letting go of his hatred for his father. Somehow it seemed to keep him going, even though he was going nowhere.

He denied his anger was eating him up and making his body, as well as his relationships, even sicker. Andrew continued hating his father, and the hatred continued destroying Andrew.

Step Six and HIV Infection

It's been said many times that resentment toward others hurts only us, not the people, places, or things at which we are angry. Andrew's case exemplifies this truth, for his anger had little effect on his father, yet tore him up physically, emotionally, and spiritually. The sixth step is a tool to rid yourself of such feelings and behaviors, to enable you to progress to a fresh and peaceful feeling. With that feeling you are free to make wise choices regarding the people, places, and things in your life.

The Next Step Toward Surrender

By now you may have completed your life review (step four) and discussed it with another person (step five). Your past patterns of behavior and responses that no longer serve you might be pretty clear. Again, we are not saying it's your defects of character that produced the HIV: you are not to blame. But we are saying you can improve your situation by letting go of the faults that may be contributing to your disease or your risk of getting the disease.

Once again you are asked to make a decision to actively participate in your healing. The decision to be ready to have your character defects removed may sound simple, but it isn't. Many character defects are defense mechanisms we've built up as a result of growing up in dysfunctional families where we needed to protect ourselves from abuse and neglect. They are often deeply embedded in our psyches. Many will be afraid to give up the very things that have gotten them through life so far. But given your present circumstances, it is crucial that you do so. These defects do not work to your benefit.

Making the decision to be *willing to change* frees you to *be changed*. It releases all the negative psychic energy that drains you physically and detracts from your healing. This is a crucial step toward wholeness, as the millions who have already taken it can attest.

Step six is not something you can physically do; it requires a change of attitude. This one is an inside job. What is necessary is to become willing to change; willing to allow your Higher Self— the part of you that knows what is best for you—to change you. You can appreciate that certain acts on your part were damaging to not only your self-esteem, but to your emotions, your body, and your spirit, as well. In other words, these ways of thinking and acting did not serve your highest good.

Step four would not have been so hard to write, and step five would not have been so hard to share with another, if all your behaviors had been in your and others' best interests. You were not always expressing your Higher Self. None of us is. Nor do we suggest that any of us ever can. But it was being untrue to yourself that caused your pain. The act of letting go of these patterns can release you from this pain and bring you to a new place of healing.

Becoming Entirely Ready

All you need to do to start the ball rolling is to become entirely ready and willing to become different. What this means is to be willing to think of yourself as freed of these past habits and encumbrances, to believe you can become different. Try to see that making this step could be something positive for you. Please give yourself permission to make this step.

LINDA'S STORY

Linda knew that her relationship with Mark was unhealthy. She knew he did IV drugs and did not always agree to safe sex. He let it be known that what he did with his buddies was none of Linda's business, so any attempt on her part to influence his drug habit was out of the question. She was scared. Despite all her intellectual understanding of why she needed to break up with him, Linda panicked every time she considered ending their relationship. They'd been together for years, and she felt ill prepared to reenter the single life. She talked and cried to her friends and mother over and over again. She was finally able to imagine life without Mark, but didn't know how she would be able to tell him.

Linda finally turned to her Adult Children of Alcoholics group for help. There she learned about the sixth step and the process of becoming willing to change. She was surprised. She'd never realized there was any step between wishing to change and making the change.

Now, at a level deeper than wishing, she got ready to let go of Mark. Without feeling she could do it by herself, she became willing to let her Higher Self do it for her. At that point she could honestly say she was entirely willing to break it off with him. She felt tremendous relief. She also knew her Higher Self would soon show her how to proceed. Until she had become entirely willing, her fears had immobilized her. Once she had turned it over to her Higher Power she felt a sense of relief and knew that soon she would know how to do it. The act of willingness opened her to clearer understanding and courage, which later empowered her to leave Mark.

Doing this step means saying to yourself, Okay, I'm willing to believe that I can become different. I can say yes, yes to new ways of being that are good for me, that serve me and allow me to feel happy with myself. I make this decision! As Linda's example demonstrates, we don't need to know exactly how we will change. We simply need to open ourselves to the opportunity of change.

Surrender

Another helpful slogan is "Progress, not perfection." No human being is perfect, so you can never expect to be perfect. As the "Big Book" of AA states, "We are not saints. The point is that we are willing to grow along spiritual lines. The principles we have set down are guides to progress. We claim spiritual progress rather than spiritual perfection." You have to be able to imagine that new ways of being are possible for you: you can be flexible; you can entertain the thought that things can change for you; you have the freedom to change; and that freedom can give you a lightness and a peace beyond belief.

Fear

Whenever we think about changing something that is familiar to us, even if we know that the familiar thing is not good for us, we experience fear. This is a normal and very human response to change. It doesn't mean that we don't want to change, or that the change will not benefit us. It's merely how the brain reacts when it imagines change. Fear is an emotional and physiological response to the thought that something new is about to happen, and something familiar is about to be lost.

As a result of HIV infection or the risk for infection, you have probably experienced change more rapidly than ever before in your life. You have probably also had to consciously make more changes faster than you've ever had to make before. And you may be losing more than you've ever lost. No wonder you are afraid!

But you will be okay. Realize what the fear is telling you. It is saying that you are ready to change, ready to let go of the familiar. It may well be that avoiding fear and pain got you into many of your past predicaments. The relaxation processes in this program help you deal with the fear and work through it. Often fear is not a sign to stop, but a sign that you are ready to go forward.

How

You don't have to do it alone. Step seven explains how change takes place. Right now, all you have to do is change your attitude, and surrender yourself to a Power greater than yourself. It is the same Higher Power you turned your will and your life over to in step three. That Power will change you. Because you can be changed only if you are willing, the attitude of surrendering to change is very important. You must become entirely ready and willing to change before you can go on to step seven, where the change actually starts to occur.

Where to Start

We all resist change. If we didn't, we would have changed long ago. Don't be hard on yourself for initially resisting, and don't worry about changing all of your behaviors at once. Just start with those behaviors, or ways of responding, that caused you the most pain in step four.

It's hard to imagine myself different. I've been this way for so long, you may say. That's okay. No one takes this step without feeling fear. You'll be fine. Several million people in AA and other twelve-step programs have done it, and every one of them was afraid. What do you have to lose? Probably only a lifetime of guilt and awful feelings about yourself.

"Will I become a shell of my former self?" No, but it sure may feel like it in the beginning. You will become more your authentic self, more like who you have always been capable of being; who you always have been inside. You will find yourself acting more like the ideal self you have always imagined yourself to be or wished you were. In time you will find that some of the things that feel like losses now are replaced with much healthier ways of being. But that may be hard to imagine now. These new responses and behaviors may feel a little strange for a while, but you will become much more comfortable with them as time goes on.

You don't need those old ways of acting and thinking; saying you do is just the disease of addiction talking. People don't become addicted only to chemicals, but also to ways of acting and thinking.

These patterns are often ingrained in the psyche; in order to break them, you must be careful of patterns of denial, which can entrap you.

You will eventually become accustomed to approaching the world as your true self, with new behaviors and responses that feel nurturing and comforting to you. You will be coming from your Higher Self more and more often, enjoying the security that brings.

"Let Go and Let God"

Often it is the very thing that you resist that seems to persist. When you consistently mentally beat yourself up over something, you unknowingly deepen the impression of the act in your mind. You are unconsciously practicing the very thing you want to avoid. And the impression of what you don't want to happen becomes stronger and stronger. Therefore the next time the situation comes up you may act on what you have learned: you may do exactly what you practiced in your mind.

You don't want to memorize things that you don't want to do! That's why mentally beating yourself up is self-defeating. Instead, stop the mental picture and replace it with the picture of how you want to be and act. Once that positive picture is in your mind, relax. Don't try so hard. "Let go and let God." Become willing to let your Higher Power do the rest of the work.

Positive Self-Talk: Becoming Ready

Just as negative self-talk keeps you stuck, positive statements initiate change in you. The more you use them, the more you solidify your desired changes.

- I am making a decision to become ready and willing to let go of my worst behaviors.

- I am learning to act, speak, feel, and think in a different way: a way that serves me, not one that destroys me.

- I am becoming entirely ready to have myself be changed.

- I will surrender all of my old self-defeating patterns of behavior and open myself to change.

First Things First: An Exercise

You can start by writing down the three behaviors and three attitudes that have been harming you. Go slowly and work first with the things that are causing the most harm. "First Things First."

JAMES'S STORY

James quit doing drugs, drinking alcohol, smoking cigarettes, and eating meat all at once. In addition, he started working out two hours each day, and changed his job, his relationship, and his residence. Within two months the strain got to him. Depleted, tired, and unfulfilled, he was again doing drugs and drinking (which led to his engaging in unsafe sex). He was so discouraged about his relapse that he just became bitter, gave up, and went back to his old way of life.

Easy Does It

Be kind to yourself. These patterns took a long time to develop, and you can't change everything overnight. This is a lifetime process, and you will come back to this step over and over again as you change and release more unwanted patterns. You can't work on all of them at the same time. Work on the three that are doing you the most harm right now. You know what they are.

Engaging in unsafe sex, using drugs, and drinking alcohol are the three most destructive behaviors you could do, and if you are practicing any or all of these, they must be addressed immediately. If James had tried to change the sex, drugs, and alcohol he might have had a chance to change the other things later. With the drugs and alcohol out of his system he would have had a chance to change his attitudes. He tried to change too many things too fast; he ended up feeling overwhelmed and changing nothing.

Mental Rehearsal: Relaxation

In your mind's eye see your three most self-destructive behaviors and the accompanying three attitudes clearly. Become willing to give them up, become willing to be different, and become willing to allow your Higher Self to express itself physically, mentally, emotionally, and spiritually. Become willing to move toward health rather than disease. You may wish to repeat over and over to yourself, until it feels true, that you are willing to change each behavior and attitude.

After you have written down these six things about yourself and are willing to change, do the "Imagery for Letting Go" in Chapter 4. These relaxation processes are designed to assist you in dealing with the fear, sadness, and loss associated with change. They help you to relax so that you can entertain the possibility of change with greater ease.

Once you are deeply relaxed, imagine enacting the behaviors you are now willing to change. Then imagine yourself behaving differently, the way your Higher Self would. Mentally practice behaving differently. Imagine putting your old, worn-out behaviors into a special box and sending them to your Higher Power. Surrender that part of yourself to your Higher Power, as Linda did in the earlier example. Imagine yourself free and unburdened: new.

Sixth-Step Affirmations

Today I surrender all of my past behaviors that have harmed me or others.

Today I realize that I can change in spite of my fear of changing.

Today I know that through change I will feel peace.

Today I know that change will heal me.

Today I am at peace with myself and the world.

SEVEN

Opening to The Healing Power

STEP SEVEN
HUMBLY ASKED the GOD of our understanding to REMOVE our SHORTCOMINGS

HUMBLY *without vanity; meekly; without pretense*

ASKED *inquired or sought by request*

GOD *Higher Power, any positive force you believe to be more powerful than yourself*

REMOVE *to take away; to cause to leave*

SHORTCOMINGS *deficiencies or flaws*

The sixth step asked you to become willing to be different. The philosophy of step seven asks for action. It can assist you in tapping into the strength and wisdom of your Higher Power as you surrender your character defects and allow this Power to change you.

TIM'S STORY

Tim realized that his drinking and using drugs were detrimental to his health. At the clinic, when he was counseled on his HIV antibody status, he was told that stopping was critical. He also knew that when he had unsafe sex he was usually "wiped out," not sufficiently aware to protect himself or his partners. After finding out he was infected with HIV, Tim was despondent for a long time. Tim was a successful businessman and maintained an expensive way of life. He thought he had finally "made it," despite his hemophilia, and was bitter about this sudden turn of events. He figured his willpower could help him avoid using mind-altering chemicals if he just tried hard enough.

He discovered that he could stay away from drugs and alcohol for weeks and months on end, but would eventually end up loaded. Alice, his wife of several years, insisted that he use condoms most of the time, but when Tim was drunk he became so belligerent she would just give in and allow him to have unsafe sex with her. She was also frustrated and upset when Tim would end up staying out all night after another binge. His binges seemed to be getting closer and closer together since he had found out about his antibody status. Alice repeatedly asked him to get help, and left brochures describing various treatment centers and clinics around the house. But Tim refused to go for help or to attend the support groups for HIV-positive hemophiliacs and their families at the local Hemophilia Foundation chapter. He said that he had to drink socially, his clients expected it, and it was Alice's problem, not his.

He was becoming abusive when drinking, so Alice started attending Al-Anon meetings and threatened to leave. Tim knew about treatment centers and he knew about AA, but insisted he could handle it on his own and certainly didn't need "anyone's pity or sloppy sentimentality."

Tim developed a severe pain in his abdomen and was afraid he had an HIV-related condition. While he was in the hospital pancreatitis was diagnosed. The pain was excruciating. The doctor explained to Tim that the pancreatitis was not related to HIV, but was from his drinking. Any more drinking would bring on another attack; and drinking was no longer a choice. He had to stop.

When Tim got home he and Alice had a long talk. Tim was more depressed than Alice had ever seen him. "I don't think you understand, Alice; I don't want to live if I have to stop drinking." "That's the most ridiculous thing I've ever heard," said Alice. "A lot of people don't drink. That's just a lame excuse."

"I'm not a lot of people. I can't talk to my clients without a few drinks. How do you think we got this house and that fancy car, for Christ's sake! And don't even start on me about a treatment center or AA. I don't think I can stop. And I don't want to stop. Can't you hear me!"

On Father's Day Tim woke up, probably again ashamed of what he had done the night before, and probably in a great deal of physical as well as psychic pain. Alice was at her sister's with the kids. His business partner found him early in the afternoon. Half a bottle of scotch, an empty Valium bottle, and a gun were at his side. A huge hole was in the back of Tim's head.

Tim could not break through the denial of his alcoholism or his HIV infection. His failure to do so resulted in his increasing his own risk factors as well as endangering his sexual partners. He also refused to accept the help and social support that could have prevented his severe depression. Tim's story is extreme, but not singular.

Tim could not acknowledge his own shortcomings, because his alcoholism kept him blind to himself. He was, therefore, several steps away from asking a Higher Power to remove them. Once you have accepted your reality and found a Higher Power, you are no longer alone. You are then free to honestly see yourself and turn over your character defects to your Higher Power. Unlike Tim, who unknowingly made alcohol his Higher Power and tried to escape into death, you can now escape into life, perhaps an even more precious life than you have ever known.

Step Seven and HIV Infection

In step six you became ready to have your Higher Power remove your character defects. Now in step seven you can actually ask for that change. HIV infection requires many changes, whether you are already infected and wanting to stay healthy, or are not infected and want to stay uninfected. Some changes may be easier than others. Some you may feel more willing to make than others. Any change requires a great deal of energy, but the changes required by HIV infection may require impossible amounts of energy if, like Tim, you try to make them alone on your own power. As one person put it, "I was taking AZT with one hand and drinking my vodka with the other. I was giving my body live and die messages at the same time. I knew I needed to get clear, but I wasn't sure if I could do it."

When you turn your character defects, no matter what they might be, over to your Higher Power and ask your Higher Power to remove them, your energy is freed up to do what is necessary for your healing. This way you are no longer in it alone. We are not saying that you can sit back and expect change to happen. But you can rest assured that a Power greater than you is working for removal of your shortcomings, while you take the necessary action and seek the help you need—that is to say, while you do the footwork.

Humility

Because you analyzed your life in step four, you have developed an honest appraisal of your attributes and shortcomings.

The person who thinks he or she is better than everyone else *and* the person who thinks he or she is not as good as anyone else are afflicted with the same disorder: narcissism. In reality, no one is all that good and no one is all that bad. To accept that truth is, in fact, to be humble. As a result of making a fourth-step list, you can begin to know yourself more honestly. This is an important part of what it means to be humble: being willing to accept an honest appraisal of yourself.

A great deal of humility is required to share that list with another person, which you did in step five. It takes real courage and truly demonstrates a willingness to strive for something better. Those of us who have taken a fearless moral inventory of ourselves surely know how difficult it is, but we also know, more than anyone else could know, how valuable it is. This step is based on that inventory and goes further into your emotional and spiritual healing. It provides the tools for change.

If drugs or alcohol have never been a problem for you, understand that any time we refer to quitting drugs or alcohol, you can substitute any behavior you have that you want and need to change. Any behavior can be changed using the twelve-step method; that's why the twelve-step process is so popular. But many people do have these character defects, and need to realize that not only do drugs and alcohol suppress their immune system, but they also alter their awareness and lead to other dangerous activities. Even people who haven't smoked cigarettes for years and then start smoking again often say that they had "only one cigarette" after having had a few drinks and the old habit quickly returned in full force. It is important to stop using drugs and alcohol so you have a better chance of maintaining your behavior changes.

The Process of Changing

When making any change in ourselves, we need to remember that at first we start out incompetent and unconscious: unable to live and behave as we really want and yet unaware of that. This is called denial. The first step to change is to become conscious: aware of your incompetence, aware of your shortcomings. That is the purpose of the inventory of step four. This step in the change process is accompanied by the uncomfortable feeling of watching yourself doing what you know you absolutely do not want to do. This is painful and you may become angry at yourself, but don't let these feelings overwhelm you; go easy on yourself. Try to remember that this is a natural state. It's part of the change process. For a while you will be incompetent and conscious. Only with awareness of your incompetency can any change begin. If you are able to see how you want things to be—even while you watch your old behaviors continuing—you will be motivated to make significant changes.

In the next stage you remain conscious, but now you gradually become more and more competent at these new behaviors, doing what you want to do, competently and consciously. You experience the joy of watching yourself performing the new behaviors that are your goal.

For a while, it is still very easy to slip into the old pattern. You need to be constantly vigilant to avoid sliding down that old slope.

But soon these behaviors will become true habits. You will remain competent, but act now out of your unconscious. You will automatically do what you know is right for you. You will no longer need to be perpetually focused on your new behaviors. You will be competent and unconscious: automatically doing what you know to be the right thing.

You can then go on to change other behaviors and attitudes in the same way. First bring them into your awareness, and start the whole process over on a different set of patterns you wish to change. The use of imagery is most helpful during this stage. When you are deeply relaxed, mentally rehearse how you want to do things. This will reinforce and quicken the change in your unconscious.

ALBERT'S STORY

Albert had been using drugs and alcohol since he was fourteen. He had been using IV drugs on and off for the past ten years. It was just a normal part of life. Nearly everyone in his neighborhood and his family used one thing or another.

When the AIDS scare hit, Albert thought it was just a big scam. He didn't know anyone who was sick, and he knew plenty of people who shot drugs. He talked to an outreach worker who was passing out bleach and condoms. He really liked the guy and vaguely remembered him from when he was just a kid. From what Albert could remember, he had been a serious dope fiend. He seemed sincere enough, and was serious about people cleaning their works and using condoms. But Albert still felt dubious.

As time went on, one friend of Albert's after another got sick. They all said it was the flu or pneumonia, but as they got sicker and sicker everyone knew that it wasn't just the flu or pneumonia. Albert thought there might really be something to this AIDS business after all.

His "old lady" had been on his back about the drugs for a long time. Now she was starting to talk to him about using condoms and cleaning his works. Albert was enraged! This AIDS "shit" was really making life complicated.

But Albert was finding that scoring wasn't pleasurable like it used to be. He was worried about AIDS, but he didn't know if he could stop the drugs. He'd gone on methadone once before after a bad dose, but hadn't stayed clean for long. He decided to give it another try, but this time he decided to go to a Narcotics Anonymous meeting like the worker at the health clinic had said to do. This guy said once Albert linked up with a Higher Power it would help remove his need for drugs.

It sounded pretty wild to Albert, but he figured he didn't have much to lose at this point. He'd rather be dead than be as sick as some of his friends, and he was tired of having his old lady on his back. He started going to NA meetings while he was on the waiting list for the methadone clinic. He stopped going to the shooting galleries and started cleaning his works. He figured he was doing the footwork and would give this Higher Power "shit" a try. If it could remove his craving to use, it sure would have to be a "Higher" Power!

Albert, unlike Tim, was able to face up to his drug problem. Armed with this awareness he took some active steps toward his healing. The previous steps invited you to become more aware. Now step seven challenges you to use that awareness for positive change. Unfortunately, change does not come easily. That's why the concept of a Higher Power described in detail in steps two and three is so important. Albert did what he needed to do, and, supported by a willingness to believe in a Higher Power, he was given the strength that is born from faith.

Positive Self-Talk: Wanting to Be Different

- I want to be different in certain areas, and I can and will be different.

- I no longer try to avoid pain by using people, places, or things to fill the emptiness inside me.

- I now choose to work through and learn from the pain, rather than run from it.

- I now seek joy in ways that serve others and myself.

- I am learning to respect others and myself.

- My Higher Power can give me the courage to change.

Easy Does It

Remember, as always, "Easy does it." You deserve to treat yourself with compassion and patience. In this world of confusion and stress, you may find that even though you are making progress, sometimes you slip back into old behaviors. But, as we have mentioned before, any system tends to resist change. When you get distracted, or are under a great deal of stress, old behaviors may resurface. That happens to all humans. It only means you have to be more vigilant at those times and make a more concerted effort to turn over to your Higher Power whatever it is you are trying to change, and let your Higher Power deal with the problem. Then you need to take action, to do the footwork. You do the work and leave the outcome to your Higher Power. In so doing, you can feel empowered by taking care of the tasks at hand and yet relieved of fear and worry, because you have a stronger Force working behind the scenes.

You Have What You Need in Order to Change

All that is necessary for change is an initial awareness of what you need to change. You probably already have that awareness; you know what you want to change. *Some changes need to happen first.* If, for example, you engage in anything other than safe sex, you must change that immediately, because it puts you and others in the most danger.

Drugs and alcohol are next. If you find that you cannot go without drinking or using drugs, you need to either get treatment and/or go to AA or Narcotics Anonymous.

If you are not dealing with these specific character defects, you can use this seventh step on whatever character defect stands between you and others, stands between you and your own happiness. It could be dishonesty or pride or jealousy. You may be trying to control others and, in so doing, actually driving them away. Anything that you don't want to be doing anymore is appropriate. Most people draw upon the inventory they made in the fourth step to help them decide what character defects they have.

A Very Special Shortcoming: Relapse

It is important to remember that we are dealing with chronic situations. Habitual ways of expressing sexuality are chronic. Drug use and alcohol abuse are chronic. Codependent or controlling ways of interacting with others are chronic. All behaviors you use to run away from the pain in your life are all part of a chronic condition.

The hallmark of a chronic condition is that it often involves relapse, meaning that you may revert to old behavior. This is a built-in shortcoming that you may have.

If you find that you already have relapsed in any area or if you should relapse in the future, forgive yourself and come back to this step and again ask your Higher Power to remove this shortcoming. Don't waste even a second beating yourself up with guilt, shoulds, or should nots. If relapse was not part of these chronic conditions, there would never have been a need for Alcoholics Anonymous or any other twelve-step program.

Examine what you think may have led to your relapse so that you can learn from your experience and avoid similar situations in the future. Let's say your relapse was with alcohol; in order to meet people you were going to bars, where you ended up drinking. Now you need to find a new place to meet people. A bar is a slippery place for someone who is trying not to drink alcohol. Give yourself a break; don't make it harder by placing temptation right in front of yourself.

> *Albert was doing fine until his cousin came to visit for the holidays. He had been on methadone for a few weeks and was even attending a NA meeting for methadone users. But when he wanted to celebrate with his cousin he found himself shooting up again. Albert soon realized how delicate his commitment to himself was. He understood the phrase about drugs and alcohol being "cunning, baffling, and powerful." It was as if he had never stopped. He was encouraged by the people at the meeting to just let go of his relapse and start over again, "one day at a time." Albert hopes that he learned something from his relapse. He believes that a relapse is bad only if he doesn't learn from it, and he thinks he learned how very fragile his newly found way of life really is.*

If your relapses are usually sexual you may want to become involved in twelve-step programs specifically for sexual issues. There are several different groups, including Sex Addicts Anonymous and Sex and Love Addicts Anonymous.

Codependency and Abuse as Relapse Dynamics

Some people have a hard time maintaining behavior change because of codependency or previous abuse issues. Most of the people we have talked to who are infected with HIV have problems with codependency needs. People who are codependent live their lives through others and have many problems in relationships. They tend to use others as the source of their identity, value, and well-being. As a result, they have difficulty with boundaries: where they leave off and where others start. They are easily influenced and are often passive-aggressive or submissive. It is hard for them to stick up for themselves, to say no. They have severe problems with intimacy and trust, as well as maintaining their own sense of reality. Not being able to assert yourself and demand safe sex or refuse drugs is an example of codependency.

People who come from families where there was an addiction, such as alcohol, drugs, food, or gambling, or from families where one of the parents had a chronic illness, or from families where there was physical, sexual, emotional, or mental abuse, or rigid, profound religious beliefs, or the premature death of a parent, often develop the characteristics of codependency. They are "adult children" because they did not mature emotionally, owing to their inadequate emotional nurturing as children. On the other hand, people from homes where there were none of these problems can also develop strong codependency traits.

There are twelve-step programs for people with codependency needs, as well as counselors who specialize in this field. There are also many good books on the subject. Al-Anon meetings are very useful; we strongly recommend that you attend them for at least six months before starting into any other twelve-step programs, such as Adult Children of Alcoholics (ACOA) (or other dysfunctional families) or Codependents Anonymous (CODA) for this specific issue. If your relapses are with drugs or alcohol, these groups are not meant to replace AA or NA. They are just additional supports.

Following is a modified list of the characteristics of a co-dependent, read at some ACOA meetings. Read through the list and notice what statements feel familiar. If you find these descriptions fit you, you may need to get support in this area and look at some old abuse patterns you have developed along the way. These may be interfering with your life now.

1. We have low self-esteem and feel inadequate. We fear discovery of the real us will cause rejection.

2. We fear rejection and disapproval. We react by creating characters that are acceptable to others.

3. At times our identities seem to wander without conviction or direction. We often feel independent, alone, or unique.

4. We cannot easily trust in loved ones, peers, or authority figures. We don't know how. We don't really trust ourselves.

5. We grieve for the families we never had. (This may not be conscious, but we may find ourselves "adopting" others and calling them Mom or Dad.)

6. We become compulsive and obsessive in our behaviors.

7. We gravitate to people we feel need us. We lose those people when they outgrow their need for us. Our feelings of inadequacy are hidden in positions of superiority.

8. We associate anger with violence and rejection, and are afraid of expressing strong feelings and losing control. We believe that showing feelings is a weakness.

9. We learned how to live with stress in childhood and unknowingly try to recreate the chaotic way of life with which we are familiar.

10. We make excuses for others' weaknesses and have unreasonable expectations for ourselves and society at large.

11. We are afraid to reveal our secrets for fear of rejection or disapproval.

12. We are unable to let go, relax, and have fun.

13. We are afraid of intimacy and have difficulty forming close relationships.

14. We are unable to ask for what we want or what we need.

15. We withdraw from others and isolate ourselves when we experience the pain of friendships.

16. We are hypersensitive to the needs of others.

17. We have difficulty hearing positive statements and are critical of ourselves and others.

18. We build up barriers to protect ourselves from our own insecurities.

19. We become aware of feelings that seem to separate us from others, and we find ourselves depressed.

Dr. Jan Kennedy, in her book *Touch of Silence: A Healing from the Heart*, addresses people who have been abused. If you have been abused or treated cruelly, it may be helpful for you to read what she has said about what happens to the abuse victim. *People who did not suffer abuse do not have these characteristics.* If you do not remember being abused and yet identify with many of the statements, you can assume that you probably were at some time, in some way, abused. It is common for people who have been abused to have no memory of the abuse. Your mind may have repressed the memory in an attempt to protect you.

This list is merely to give you some understanding so that you can be more gentle with yourself. If you have ever wondered whether you were crazy because of some of the feelings discussed in the list that follows, let us assure you that you are not. This is just what happens to people who have been abused. You are not crazy!

Behaviors and Attitudes That Result from Abuse

1. Someone approaches you sexually in a normal, healthy way, and you feel you have no right to say no or you can't say no. You have feelings of frustration and guilt for not having better control over your behavior, and you feel as if you should.

2. Whenever someone comes to you with a hard luck story, you do your best to make things better for that person. Regardless of the situation, you may feel ultraresponsible, as if it's all your fault. You continually feel that you're to blame when bad things happen.

3. You have feelings of guilt whenever you put yourself first. It's as if you owe other people for your right to exist. You feel obligated to comply with what others say you should or shouldn't do.

4. You have feelings of low self-worth, as if everyone else is better, more important, smarter, stronger, or has more authority than you do. You don't trust your inner guidance about what's best for you.

5. You feel like insignificant trash, ugly, lazy, stupid, fat, inarticulate, and downright no good. You feel shame, embarrassment, rage, and depression.

6. "If I make it up and stick with it, then it'll be real." You trust your fantasies and dreams more than what seems to be real. Magical thinking or mind-body separation can lead to dissociative states, blackouts, and totally weird behavior.

7. "I'll teach others how to behave just like me and be nice like I am." You work to get agreement for your behavior so you won't feel so isolated and alone, and if others act like you, it must be okay. This sets up urges for control, gangup, and "us against them." You have feelings of aggression and defense.

8. "I'm less than, therefore I deserve (for example, to be treated the way people treat me, to be poor, to always obey and never think for myself)." You have feelings of defeat. You adjust your behavior and attitudes to accommodate what others have said about you. You experience loss of your willpower, spirit, will to live, creativity, and willingness to risk, and are basically just marking time until you die, and surviving the best you can.

If you really fit these descriptions you would benefit from some counseling. Again, even if you are not infected, these issues can impede your healing and your health. Everyone can benefit from a seventh step on codependency, but depending on how severe your issues are, counseling may be your indicated footwork.

"Humbly Asked the God of Our Understanding to Remove Our Shortcomings"

Now, if you wish, is the time to surrender yourself to that Power and let it change you. Let go and let your Higher Power do the work. "Let go and let God!" You can ask in a prayer or you can ask in just plain words. All you need to do is humbly ask.

"Turn it over" is another AA slogan. It means turn everything over to your Higher Power, even your character defects, the things you want to change about yourself. That way you don't have to struggle so hard. "*I can't.* My Higher Power *can.* I think I'll let it/him/her" is another phrase twelve-steppers use when referring to something with which they have been having trouble. Like Albert, you can turn it over to your Higher Power.

Having turned your defects over to your Higher Power, you may become aware of opportunities that arise to work on these defects. Say, for example, one of your shortcomings is that you have little patience. One day you may find yourself in a line at a bank, and the person in front of you is taking a terrifically long time, asking the teller many questions, making mistakes, chit-chatting. You may begin to feel angry and impatient. This is a perfect opportunity to thank your Higher Power for a chance to grow, a chance to work on your patience. Once you turn things over to your Higher Power, it will not simply erase your short-comings, but will instead grant you opportunities to change. This is your Higher Power's gift to you, and you show your appreciation in the way you use these situations to further your personal growth.

Positive Self-Talk: Asking

- I humbly ask now, with full expectation that my Higher Power will help me.

- I allow my Higher Power to change me, and I am changed.

- Even though I may not be aware of it, the change is happening at this very moment.

- I can stop trying so hard, and I can let go and let God.

- Soon my behaviors and my thoughts will prove to me that I am changed.

- I now act more and more out of my Higher Self.

Seventh-Step Prayer

Here is the prayer that AA members say when taking the seventh step.

> My Creator, I am now willing that you should have all of me, good and bad. I pray that you now remove from me every single defect of character which stands in the way of my usefulness to you and my fellows. Grant me strength, as I go out from here, to do your bidding.

Many people in twelve-step programs say this prayer every day, along with the third-step prayer (on page 97) as part of their daily program.

Image Rehearsal for Writing Your Own Script

Take some time to do the following relaxation process. The longer script is on page 298. Imagine yourself doing things differently, and see the change coming over you like a healing blanket of light. This experience will give you an opportunity to increase your awareness of your emotional potential, and to become more sensitive to the range and subtlety of your feelings. It will also teach you to trust your feelings, to balance them, and to use your emotional state as an important guide in making decisions and choices in your life, especially those involving your wellness.

Part 1: Deep Relaxation

Part 2: Image Rehearsal

Take a deep breath in and, as you let it out, imagine you're a balloon letting out all the air, becoming completely flat and relaxed. Imagine with each breath out that loving light is being breathed out like a mist and that this mist is visible. It is taking a physical shape in front of you, forming an image of you looking and feeling the way you'd like to look and feel: healthy, strong, and serene.

With each breath in, breathe this image into your body. Notice the feelings in your chest and upper abdomen, without attempting to name your emotions. Sometimes they may be calm and un-ruffled, like a peaceful lake. Don't attempt to change how you feel; just accept it.

With each breath out, repeat each phrase silently.

- I can allow myself to be at peace.

- I open myself to joy and happiness.

- I can choose to let go of attachments to ideas.

- I have learned to calm my emotions at will.

- I feel confidence and strength from within.

- I can assert myself and be expressive.

- My Higher Power gives me the strength to resist any negative influence.

Imagine yourself now in the kind of situation that might have been difficult for you to handle in the past. But you are different now, and you will handle it differently. Feel yourself making the correct choices, writing your own script.

Repeat this process for several other challenging events that might occur in your future. Each time you use your imagination in this way, you are reinforcing the image and outcome that you want.

Part 3: Reawakening

Allow yourself to come to full wakefulness or, if you wish, let yourself rest or go to sleep.

Seventh-Step Affirmations

Today I can humbly ask my Higher Power to relieve me of my shortcomings.

Today I am able to ask my Higher Power for assistance.

Today I take time to thank my Higher Power for making these changes possible.

Today I feel relief and go forward with the conviction that I am changed for the better.

Today I am at peace with myself and the world.

EIGHT

Willing to Mend

STEP EIGHT
MADE a LIST of all persons we had HARMED and BECAME WILLING to make AMENDS to them all

---

MADE *created; caused to exist*

LIST *a record of names*

HARMED *hurt or injured; damaged*

BECAME *passed from one state to another; grew; changed*

WILLING *having the mind inclined; desirous*

AMENDS *compensation for harm done*

Step Eight can allow forgiveness to start healing your heart. Just by being willing to mend relationships, you can feel a burden lifted. You can learn how releasing strained relationships frees up your energy to deal with your daily living and daily healing.

ANNETTE'S STORY

Annette thought the eighth step was the most absurd step of all. She hated her mother, "and with good reason." Her mother had deserted Annette and her three brothers when Annette was very young. Annette had had to give up her dreams of graduating from school in order to stay home and care for her brothers. "Be willing to make amends to her?

Never!" Within a short time Annette continued to get sicker and weaker and found it very hard to deal with the many additional burdens HIV infection brought into her life.

Finally, after much counseling, Annette realized the bitter resentment she felt toward her mother was only hurting her. It affected her in ways she had not realized. She thought by just not seeing or talking to her mother she had put her out of her life. In fact, Annette discovered many subtle ways this unfinished business with her mother robbed her of vital energy. This was energy she needed to be who she wanted to be and to do what she wanted to do. She came to see how in her daily activities this emotional parasite was damaging her precious spirit, as an internal physical parasite might insidiously feed upon and damage her body. And she needed this spirit to be as free and clear as possible to help her deal with her infection.

She called her buddy and said she was ready to work an eighth step on her relationship with her mother. She was willing to make whatever amends she needed to make, even to her mother, if it would help her feel better and more peaceful inside. After hanging up the phone, Annette already began to feel the sense of relief that comes from willingness alone. She could hardly believe it.

The Social Beings that We Are

Steps eight and nine have to do with relationships. As human beings we are social by nature. It is through relationships that we discover who we are. They make us whole and give life an added dimension and meaning. Have you ever noticed how commonly people introduce themselves by referring to important relationships: daughter or son of, sister or brother of, mother or father of, lover, wife, or husband of?

Studies have shown that human beings deprived of social contacts fail to thrive, and may even die of loneliness. Long-term epidemiologic studies indicate that people who are single, separated, divorced, or widowed are two to three times more likely to die than their peers and are hospitalized for mental disorders five to ten times more frequently. Widowers are especially hard hit, as they are hospitalized three times more often for infections and have three times the death rate of their peers. Medical students with higher loneliness scales had decreased natural killer cell (an immune system cell) activity, and a twenty-year study of medical students showed that students who lacked close parental relationships were more likely to develop various forms of cancer in their adulthood.

Relationships also affect the health of pregnant women and the outcome of their pregnancy. One study shows that 75 percent of mothers without support developed complications such as fetal distress, stillbirth, cesarean sections, and induced labor. Only 12 percent of the mothers with support developed these complications. In uncomplicated labors, the mothers who had someone close to them there to support them had labors lasting only half as long as mothers who didn't. Psychoneuroimmunologists suspect the chemicals produced by prolonged feelings of loneliness and fear in some way account for these statistics. Even though we may not understand electricity, we know how to turn on the lights. Likewise, even though we may not yet understand exactly *how* relationships affect our health, we do know that they *do*. And we do know that the healthier your relationships are, the better chances you have with any disease, including HIV infection.

Step Eight and HIV Infection

Whether you are already infected or trying to avoid becoming infected, it is difficult to be whole and healed unless your relationships are completed. If you have any unresolved relationships, you have unfinished business. Now is the time for healing, at least your part of the relationships. These relationships are like open, oozing wounds, and will continue to drain you of your life's blood and energy.

To bring your best to life, you need all your energy. It is important to know you have done everything that you can to help heal every area of your life, including the emotional areas.

You need to be free of any guilt you may still feel for ways in which you thought, felt, or acted, that failed to serve your higher good or that of others. You can feel the freedom of release that comes when you are able to forgive others, as well as yourself. The fourth step is an excellent beginning. Steps eight and nine can help you gain more insight into your ways of relating, and assist you in healing any wounded relationships.

Reviewing Your List

If you wrote a fourth step, it is helpful to look at the list of people you named. If you've lost it, you can just start a new one; don't worry, you'll remember the names. Starting with this list, add anyone else who comes to mind. When you are finished, you will have the names of all the people, dead and alive, whom you have harmed, or who have harmed you in any way: physically, mentally, emotionally, or spiritually. The reason you need to include people who have harmed you is so you can explore the effects of that damage and work toward forgiveness of it.

When you think of *any* person and get an uncomfortable feeling or twinge in your heart or your gut, that person's name needs to be on your eighth-step list. That includes anyone with whom you did not keep the Golden Rule—"Do unto others as you would have them do unto you"—or who did not keep the rule with you. These are the people who still live rent free inside you. There they reside, keeping your gut in knots and your heart in spasm. You may have become numb to the pain over the years, but it is there nonetheless. The chemicals of anger, fear, and loneliness silently eat away at your immune cells and your peace of mind; starting this list is like writing their eviction notices.

The easiest way to do step eight is to jot down next to the names of these people some words or phrases that bring to mind the difficulty you experienced in these relationships. Writing approximate dates is helpful. Remember to include parents, brothers, sisters, children, co-workers, friends, lovers, and acquaintances. You may have forgotten some of their names, and some you may never have known. That's okay. Try to write down something that at least identifies them to you.

But She Owes Me the Apology

When children are reprimanded they often say, "But she hit me first!" What the parent or teacher usually says is "Two wrongs don't make a right." It's amazing how long it takes some of us to learn that. If you haven't learned it yet, it's important to understand it now.

It's critical that your list include people who may have wronged you, even people whose wrongs may have been much greater to you than yours to them. The point of this step is that you become willing to accept responsibility for your part in every relationship, no matter who was the bigger "bad guy." This is probably the hardest part for all of us. Your ego may cry out, "But if he hadn't _____, then I wouldn't have _____!" Even if the only negative response from you was in reaction to a much greater offense, it is still important to look at your response.

Why? Because it is you who lives in your skin. And it is you who wants to feel good about living there. Anything about yourself in relationships that keeps you from feeling completely clean and whole needs to be addressed. If not, these things will drain your energy and leave you weakened and inclined to act in ways that are harmful to you and perhaps others. Encourage yourself to take this opportunity to look at the part you played in every soiled relationship. The work that is suggested is for your peace of mind and physical well-being. Blaming and justifying, although completely understandable, won't be of any help in this process.

Even if every court in the land would find you justified, if you can let go of that kind of thinking, you can clearly see your part. Then you will be able to mend and forgive. You are responsible for *only* your part in any situation, even if you were blamed for more. Another's part is another's responsibility. This is only *your* list. You are the one who is trying to grow and heal. If you wish, you can pray that the other person too will come to see what he or she needs to let go. Indeed, the other person may need healing too, but you can take responsibility for only yourself. The other person is responsible for his or her own healing, if he or she chooses to become healed.

171

Forgiveness

In order for you to accept your part in all of this, however, it is vital to have an attitude of willingness. Just *consider* the possibility of forgiving the other person. This is an attitude step, not an action step. All you have to do is try to keep an open mind. "Forgive that jerk? Are you kidding me!" may be your first response. The biggest reason for forgiving the other person is really quite selfish. Any anger or resentment you hold toward another hurts you, emotionally and physically. It keeps your body riled up and wastes your valuable energy. HIV infection can have the effect of helping you keep your priorities clear. You *need* to have all your energy available to you to either prevent or deal with the infection.

Of all the internal actions you can take regarding your attitude toward another person, and, indeed, toward yourself, there is none quite as empowering as forgiveness. You may need to think of that other person as sick, emotionally, mentally, or spiritually. It is easier to consider forgiving a sick person, and, for sure, anyone who abuses another is certainly sick.

Dealing with Past Abuse

If you were abused as a child you may have a very hard time here. This is why we suggest you have a counselor who can help you through childhood issues. There are several methods used to work through issues of abuse. Plese refer to "Codependency and Abuse as Relapse Dynamics" in Chapter 7 for further understanding of the dynamics of abuse and how it may have affected you.

These exercises may sound harsh at first. But there is method to this madness. Most of us have minimized our suffering and the effect other people have had on our lives and our spiritual well-being. Even though you may not consciously feel like you were affected, you were. Unless you experience the feelings, they stay stuck inside you, coming out in self-defeating ways that can be harmful to others and yourself. You may have medicated these feelings for years with drugs, alcohol, food, relationships, sex, or work. But medicating feelings never gets rid of them. They only go deeper and often come out in unpredictable ways. You may have found yourself reacting to someone or something in a way that appeared to be inappropriate. For example, someone pulls in front of your car and you feel a strong desire to kill that person. This desire is undoubtedly anger coming up after years of denial or self-medication. When this happens it leaves you, as well as the target of these feelings, confused.

Now is a good time to drain the well. Those old feelings smell and they contaminate your precious inner spirit. They've been in there too long. If you are not willing to get them out in a controlled fashion—in the ways we describe or the ways your therapist suggests—they will sneak out when you least expect them. You might start feeling out of control and bad about yourself. We all act inappropriately sometimes, but the sooner you start emptying the well, the sooner you will behave as your Higher Self more often.

The following are just two techniques. If these work for you, great. If another works better, we encourage you to use it. But find a gentle and controlled way to empty your well, so something fresh can refill it.

One method that a therapist who treats abused people recommends is imagining the abuser gets punished in whatever way you want and feel is appropriate. Let it be as physical and awful as you want. Let your imagination run free and without judgment, remembering that this is not *really* happening to the abuser. Cry and yell out loud anything and everything you have ever wanted to say as you imagine the abuser sitting in an empty chair in front of you. Feel the vitality of that anger. Be specific in your out-pourings to the abuser. Let him or her know *exactly* what you've felt all these years. Express how this has affected you. When you have vented all of your anger and grief, try to imagine him or her adequately punished in whatever graphic way works for you. See the abuser begging for your forgiveness and groveling at your feet.

Next try imagining yourself reluctantly and patronizingly accepting this person's apology as he or she pleads with you for forgiveness. When you are ready, which may take some time, move to the place of seeing this person as sick and feeling sadness for yourself and sadness for him or her. Let your cleansing tears wash over you. Hear your cries of anguish. When you are tired from the release, end by praying for that person and for your own spiritual healing.

Another effective method is one used by a gay priest who is a recovering alcoholic and a therapist. He asks his clients to kneel before going to bed at night and talk or pray to their Higher Power in this way: "I want you to punish that asshole really bad. I want _____ to suffer slow and long. I want you to bring _____ to his or her rotten knees in really intense pain. I want you to have _____ lose everything (he or she) has ever held dear, while I watch. I want to see _____ writhing in pain. I want to see _____ screaming for mercy."

Pray like this every night until you are exhausted with this kind of thinking and praying. It may take days or weeks to get to this point. You'll find in time that your prayer shifts to one that may go like this: "Okay, Higher Power, I think _____ has been punished enough. Now I want to see _____ begging me for forgiveness. I want _____ crawling in agony over the realization of what the jerk has done. I want to stand over _____ while (he or she) kneels at my feet and begs for forgiveness, and I want to say 'No! You asshole, suffer some more!' "

You may have to stay with this kind of prayer for a while. When you become tired of this kind of prayer you will find yourself sliding into, "Higher Power, I know _____ is sick and I know I'm sick. Please help us both. We need it so badly."

Moving through such a series of emotions and perspectives takes some time, but progress will come. Joining a support group, such as Adult Children of Alcoholics, can help.

One thing we know from the study of abusive people is that most people who abuse others were themselves abused as children. That certainly doesn't make it right or make the pain they inflict on others any less, but it may give you some understanding. The knowledge of this fact may make it easier for you to forgive that person. It may also help you understand why *you* may have been abusive to others or yourself. Or you may have found yourself, as an adult, being abused in relationships and wondering why you kept picking abusive friends or lovers.

Those who were abused as children often develop abusive relationships because unconsciously they are seeking something familiar, and abuse is familiar. *Because abuse begets abuse, it is vital to deal with it.* If you can eventually forgive the person who abused you, you can discontinue this unhealthy pattern of abuse in your life. *Remember, you are not denying that the abuse occurred and you are not minimizing it. You are simply letting go of the negative way it has affected you.* You can do this by releasing the bindings that hold you to the person who abused you. Forgiveness loosens those bindings. If you don't in some way learn to forgive that person, you are giving that person the power to continue to negatively affect even your adult life.

Some therapists believe that it is useful to confront the abuser about the abuse and its impact on you. That may or may not be valuable, but step eight does not directly deal with that. We strongly suggest you have professional counseling before deciding to confront someone.

The Healing Power of Forgiveness

It seems that the attitudes we hold toward others are often the same attitudes we unconsciously hold toward ourselves. People who are judgmental and harsh with others are usually also judgmental and harsh with themselves. So once you become willing to forgive your abusers, you will become more willing to forgive yourself and begin to reconnect with yourself, and perhaps with your abusers, provided you feel safe from further abuse.

Right now it's important to allow yourself to simply consider the idea of forgiveness. You can call on your Higher Power, your Higher Self, to assist you. You may not feel very forgiving on your own. But you know that your Higher Self is big enough to forgive them. Your Higher Power can do for you that which you cannot do for yourself. It can show you the way. Your willingness to even consider the possibility of forgiveness will permit your Higher Power to take over and begin the process. You may not even want to forgive them! Part of you may even enjoy or feel you need this resentment. But it helps to remember that the only person this resentment hurts is you.

When you become willing to forgive, you can act as the highest part of yourself. When you act as your most loving part you are tapping into your wholeness. You are healing!

Positive Self-Talk: Willing to Be Willing

- Okay, okay, I will at least become willing to forgive—even though I'm not really sure I want to.

- I will think of the person who abused me as a sick person, a person who was probably abused himself or herself.

- I will feel much lighter as I consider releasing this anger and perhaps hatred.

- It's true: ultimately I benefit from forgiving others.

This is a good time to complete your list of people you have harmed and who have harmed you. You will almost always find that you respond in some unhealthy way to those who have harmed you, even if it is only resentment.

Describe the Behavior

On the list next to each person's name, describe your offensive behavior. This behavior may include lying, stealing, cheating, envying, resenting, being hostile, treating badly, gossiping, and abusing physically, emotionally, or sexually. Similarly, you may write about anyone whom you took advantage of, took moods out on, threatened, acted selfishly, irritatingly, critically, impatiently, or humorlessly toward, ignored, dominated, or passively or aggressively manipulated. This is only a partial enumeration of behaviors. You may find others that belong on your list.

Forgiving Yourself

As you look at your list, try to be gentle and forgiving of yourself. By now we hope you realize that you were always doing the best you were capable of at that moment. That was then. This is now. If you had to do it all over again, you might do it differently. You may not be able to redo the past, but you can do the next best thing. You can become *willing* to make amends for your thoughts, words, and deeds. That is all step eight suggests: to become willing.

What Are Amends?

Amends are compensation for harm done. Making amends means making an apology for any behavior that caused someone harm in any way and then making a sincere effort not to repeat that behavior. This allows you, if the person is willing, to reconnect with the damaged party. If the person is not willing or does not accept your apology, it allows you to know that you were willing and tried to reconnect with that person—and that is all that any of us can do. Even if the person won't forgive you, you know that your Higher Power has forgiven you, and you can then go on to forgive yourself. Step nine discusses this further.

Whom to Include

Make certain to include the people it may seem impossible to make amends to: the dead, the geographically distant, and the nameless people you may have harmed. It is important to become willing to make amends even to those whom you are certain would not accept your apologies. Always remember that what you are doing is for *your* healing, not theirs. Step nine will explain exactly how to go about making the amends. There is even a method for the deceased and for the nameless.

Feelings

When you are working on this step you may feel a deep sense of grief. As you think about people who may no longer be in your life because of something you did or said, you may experience feelings of sadness and remorse. Please allow yourself to feel these feelings. You needn't wallow in self-pity, but feeling the feelings is important. Grieving over your losses is important too. Let your tears wash away your feelings of sadness, and then allow yourself the freedom of knowing that today is a new day. Today you can do things differently. Today you can become willing to mend damaged relationships and let go of relationships that have damaged you. Remember that "This too shall pass." But while it's here, take a courageous deep breath and go ahead and feel it.

In order to gain the maximum benefit from the eighth and ninth steps you will want to keep your list open for any other names that come to mind. Add to your list any new names as they occur to you. Realize that it may take years before this process is complete.

Once your list is as complete as you can make it for the time being, and you have asked your Higher Self, your Higher Power, to open your heart to forgiveness, the "Imagery for Letting Go," in Chapter 4, will be helpful. When you are deeply relaxed, imagine yourself covered with a blanket of forgiveness. Give it a color, texture, and temperature. Feel it healing you. Repeat this imagery exercise at least once daily while working this step; it will keep you centered.

Allow these statements to firmly impress your mind with your willingness and intent to reconnect with others.

Eighth-Step Affirmations

Today that part of me that is pure love will make me whole.

Today that part of me that is pure love will strengthen those parts of me that have been weakened through broken and damaged relationships.

Today I am capable of forgiveness.

Today I can start to forgive others.

Today I can start to forgive myself.

Today I am willing to make the amends I know I need to make.

Today I ask my Higher Power to help me when I have difficulty considering making amends to any particular person.

Today I am at peace with myself and the world.

NINE

Reconnecting

STEP NINE
MADE DIRECT AMENDS to such people
WHEREVER POSSIBLE, EXCEPT when to do so
would INJURE them or others.

MADE *to produce*

DIRECT *straightforward; plain*

AMENDS *compensation for harm done*

WHEREVER *at whatever place*

POSSIBLE *capable of coming to pass; to be able*

EXCEPT *excluding*

INJURE *to do harm; to hurt or damage*

Step Nine is the step that can enable you to reconnect with those people, including yourself, with whom you have strained relationships. Healing these damaged relationships will also help heal your heart and spirit.

DAVID'S STORY

David's father was a hard-drinking, critical, religious zealot who emotionally, physically, and sexually abused David. As a youth David was in denial regarding the abuse and was very loyal to his dad. Then as an adult no longer in denial, David hated his father and everything for which he stood. In using the twelve steps, David began to realize that the hatred he felt for his father was really eating away at his own peace of mind and further endangering his physical health.

After working through the anger, feelings of betrayal, and deep sorrow with a counselor, David slowly became willing to forgive his father. He called his father and apologized for his part in further damaging their relationship. His father immediately started telling David how awful he, David, had been, and showed no recognition of his own misconduct. Rather than allow himself to be further abused, and acting as his own best parent, David interrupted the verbal abuse, reiterated his apology, said "Goodbye. I love you," and hung up the phone.

Several months later, when his stepmother was dying, David returned to his father and stepmother's home to help his father deal with her death. He treated his father differently than he had in the past. Instead of reacting to his past abuses David had, so to speak, switched off all the buttons. He now saw his father as a very damaged and emotionally sick human being. Because David had changed, his father's old behavior didn't trigger the same reactions. Soon he began to respond to David differently, and they were able to have an almost pleasant visit.

The peace of mind David felt after returning from his visit with his father could be seen in the spontaneity of his smile and the bounce in his walk. It was as if a tremendously heavy veil of pain had been removed. He felt freer to be himself and found his relationships with other men less strained. The energy he had used to hide the pain and stay estranged from his father was now available for David's healing work.

Step Nine and HIV Infection

Unfinished business is a constant strain. It weighs especially heavy when you are faced with a crisis, such as HIV infection. Living life to its fullest, one day at a time, is most easily done when all the pieces of your life's puzzle are together. A ninth step allows for reconnection and reconciliation with all the people in your life, even the ones with whom you have unfinished business. Step nine frees up all the emotional energy drained by damaged relationships. It gives you a way to mend that damage from your side and fit the puzzle together.

What Are Amends?

Remember, amends are not just an apology. Making amends implies a sincere attempt to change the behavior that gave rise to the need for the apology. To make an apology without a desire to be different is not making amends. Words alone are not enough. You need to be willing, like David was, to relate in a new and different way.

Do I Really Need to Make Amends?

The spirit of the ninth step suggests that you make amends. The relief of all those who have done a ninth step testifies to the remarkable value of making amends. Keep in mind that any incomplete, damaged relationship drains you of your psychic and spiritual energy. A damaged relationship is like an open wound, and your life's blood and power oozes from it.

You need and deserve total peace of mind. This is one way to get it. This is an active, kinetic step. With this action you say to your mind and to your body that you want to live. Your active pursuit of healing your relationships lets your immune system know that you are not a victim. It says that you are vital and moving toward wholeness. In return, your body can respond and also actively move toward healing.

Making Amends When You Are Truly Willing

There may be certain behaviors that you are still unwilling to change. There may even be people in your life with whom you are not ready to relate in a loving manner. If you are unable to honestly apologize for your part in a damaged relationship, and to at least be willing to relate differently, it is best to wait and make amends when you feel truly willing to forgive and be different. Please don't play games. Being dishonest and playing games are often the attitudes that helped produce the conditions you are trying to heal. Someday soon you will feel different, and when you do you can make the special amends that seem now to be impossible to make.

Repairing Broken Relationships

"To whom should I make amends first?" *No* relationship is perfect, and if you are like us, you probably have amends of some sort to make to everybody you know. The best way to start on any difficult project is to break it into small pieces and do the easy pieces first. Give yourself a break and start out with some successes.

Probably the best people to begin with are those whose names appear on your list from step eight and with whom you have a relatively good relationship, and with whom you are in touch: your friends, your co-workers, and relatives with whom you communicate frequently.

You will probably be pleasantly surprised to discover that *most* people will be quite gracious and respond positively to your sincere attempts to reconnect with them. Try starting off with something like this: "I'm working a program to help me live more comfortably and have more peace in my life. So I'd like to apologize for _____. I'll make a sincere effort to not repeat that and avoid doing anything else that would damage our relationship."

Wording and Timing

If being specific, here or at any other point in this program, is likely to be damaging to another person, be general. Use statements like, "If in any way, by my words or actions, I have harmed you, I am sorry and will try to do better in the future." Remember, the purpose of this is not to dump on anyone, stir up old embers, or inflict further pain or confusion.

It is best, therefore, to avoid being verbally specific when revealing or resurrecting the memory of any conduct on your part that would bring another further pain. Examples of this are infidelity, dishonesty, and manipulation. Making amends for this kind of behavior involves your acting differently: choosing to stop doing those things that you did in the past that would have hurt people if they had known about them.

You may be surprised to discover that most people won't even remember the event for which you are apologizing, or will respond with, "That's okay. I was just as much to blame." Some people may not even know you need to make amends to them. That's okay. They may not have been aware of how jealous or hateful you felt toward them. Again, nonspecific amends may be appropriate. You don't need to say, "I used to hate you." Gaining peace of mind at another's expense is never okay.

Also, be careful to avoid statements such as, "If you hadn't said _____, then I wouldn't have _____." The spirit of the twelve steps reminds you to look at your part, not someone else's. Remember, it is you who are making amends, not the other person. So avoid commenting on another's behavior. The purpose of the ninth step is not to get the other person to apologize to you. If the other person chooses to apologize in turn, great, but if that person doesn't, that's okay too. You have done your part to reconnect with him or her.

Also, remember that you are not the only person who is off balance and confused. Many of the people with whom you have been in relationships may have their problems too. If you think making amends to a person could cause him or her to suffer deep distress or some sort of break with reality, use your better judgment. Even though *you* may be healing, other people may be getting worse.

Try to be sensitive to the importance of timing. It is best to seek guidance from your sponsor, a friend, or a counselor in deciding when to make some amends. Not only does the ninth step require courage, it also demands prudence. Choose your timing so that it will enhance, rather than impede, the amends. Some relationships may be so volatile, or so recently damaged that you choose to wait and make amends to other people first.

It is, however, very easy to try to put off some amends indefinitely. If you are looking for total soul healing you will find that they all need to be made. Further, don't delay amends solely because of fear or embarrassment; that is not a good enough reason if you are really looking for full reconnection with yourself and others. This step requires tremendous courage. In this step your Higher Power, your Higher Self, goes to work doing for you that which you could not do for yourself.

A New Equation

It's amazing that when one person changes, the rules of the game change. Somehow this allows the entire relationship to be different. In the beginning, David's father was the same. But after David called a truce, his father also had the freedom to be different. David's allowing his Higher Self to do the acting and speaking for him seemed to encourage his father to allow his Higher Self to act and speak for him more.

If you have been estranged from your family owing to their rejection (or potential rejection) of your way of life, this can be an especially healing step for you. If your family is not too emotionally damaged, you may be surprised to find that they are very willing and able to love and accept you for who you are. Unfortunately, it is not uncommon to find that it takes a crisis to bring a family back together. A great deal of healing can come to you and your family out of this experience. Many people who have become infected have said that, in this respect, AIDS was the best thing that ever happened to them. It allowed them to reconnect with loved ones.

CARL'S STORY

I met Carl in the fall of 1986 at a support group meeting in LA. After the meeting several of the young men and I went out for something to eat and to talk. I found myself drawn to Carl, who had beautiful, soft blue eyes and a quiet manner. When it was time to leave, Carl and a few others walked me to my car. I had been watching the pain in Carl's eyes all evening.

I couldn't stand watching Carl's suffering any longer, so just as I was about to get into my car, I hugged him and asked him what was bothering him. He said, "Cindy, my parents are simple, sweet farmers in Nebraska. I just got out of the hospital with pneumonia. I am going home for Thanksgiving to tell them that I have AIDS. They don't even know I'm gay. The only one who knows is my sister. I haven't been home much since I moved here seven years ago. I feel really bad. I don't think they can take this! I feel like the character in the sick joke, 'Well, folks, the bad news is I'm gay, but the good news is I have AIDS.'

I felt truly powerless to help Carl, so I just held him, took a deep breath, and prayed for my Higher Power to talk through me. I told him that if he would practice imagining that he was home with his parents telling them that he was gay and was sick, and would imagine his mother and father coming to him and saying that they loved him and would support him no matter what, that I believed it could happen.

Stunned, Carl just looked at me and said, "Do you really believe that? Don't you think they'll go crazy?" I told him that I think we really give each other too little credit, and when the chips are down, most parents, especially mothers, will come through for their children. I then told him what had happened to me when I, eldest of three daughters and the role model for my sisters, became pregnant—right before canceling my wedding.

I was so sure that my parents would "go crazy" if I had a child out of wedlock, that I chose to attempt to kill myself rather than embarrass my very Catholic parents. Their comfort was more important to me than my own life! Obviously, despite my best attempt, I did not die and ended up going home and having to tell my parents anyway. My father did "go crazy" for a while, but my mother supported me and my father eventually came around. He was never thrilled that his first grandchild had "no father," but he lived through it. Today my daugther, who is now twenty years old and helping to edit this book, is the apple of her grandfather's eye.

I gave Carl my telephone number and asked him to call me any time he wanted. He called right after Thanksgiving to tell me that what he had been imagining was exactly what had happened. His parents had been very supportive, especially his mother.

About a year later I received a letter from Carl's mother.

Enclosed in the envelope was Carl's obituary, which she had embossed for me. She thanked me for what I had done for her son. She said that he had kept the picture of my family I sent him for Christmas and that he had spoken of me often. She thanked me over and over again and said the only thing that had bothered her was that it had taken Carl so long to come to them for support.

I am so glad I took a few minutes to speak with Carl and that I was able to allow my Higher Power to work through me. I believe that his family's response can be repeated in your life.

Hostile Relationships

Not all stories have such a happy ending, but countless similar stories are told in other twelve-step programs. These kinds of things do happen when a person becomes self-responsible, starts turning his or her will and life over to the care of his or her Higher Power, and works the steps to the best of his or her ability.

Even if you have tried before to bridge a gap with your family or others and did not find them receptive, we still suggest that you try one more time. This time use the techniques described at the end of this chapter, and see if things turn out differently.

Please don't shut down here. Finish reading before you make a judgment. Hold the "That's easy for you to say, but you don't know my family." Please keep reading and stay open-minded.

Too often when we try to apologize or make amends we slip into the "But if you hadn't . . ." routine. The minute we bring the other person's behavior into the picture, he or she becomes defensive and the whole thing goes up in the smoke of one more heated argument. This time try speaking only of yourself, with no mention of the other's behavior or actions. You will probably be surprised how differently things work out.

If you come from a home where alcoholism or substance abuse is a problem, you know the importance of timing. Take into account when this person drinks or uses drugs in determining when you will call.

Do Not Accept Abuse

The ninth step is not meant to be torture. This is a healing step so that you can feel clean and whole about at least trying to change your relationships. This is *not* an exercise in begging. If the person with whom you are trying to reconnect becomes abusive, end the conversation. If *any time* would be a bad time to call on a person, you can write a letter. This step is not meant to give anybody license to abuse you further. You have probably been abused enough by these people in your lifetime.

If old feelings of sadness for the losses you have felt or the pain you have endured come up for you, try going through the forgiveness process. Feel your feelings and cry your tears. Talk to someone or write about them, and then you will be ready to move on.

What You Are Is Not What You Did

Also remember that you are making amends for any harm or pain you have caused by your *actions:* what you did or didn't do. You are not apologizing for who you *are.* If you are homosexual and your family dislikes this, keep this in mind. If they are unwilling to accept your apology for any pain you have caused, or if the *only* pain they still feel that you have caused them is your not being who or what they want you to be, *that is their problem, not yours.* It becomes your problem only if you compound matters by not *accepting them* the way they may be, homophobia and all, or if you take responsibility for their prejudices. This may be one of the most difficult things you ever have to do. But accepting them where they are is *not* the same thing as begging or apologizing for who you are. As Bill Wilson, the cofounder of AA, says in the "Big Book" of AA, "As God's people we stand on our feet; we don't crawl before anyone!"

Having a Bad Record

If *you* are the one who has used drugs or abused alcohol, remember that the people close to you may have good reason for doubting your sincerity. They may feel that it is just one more of your many dishonesties and be reluctant to believe that you have seriously turned over a new leaf.

Some people may find it difficult or even impossible to give you yet another chance. That can be very painful, but again, this is for you. It would be nice, but it is not necessary for them to believe you. You only need to know, for yourself, that you have honestly tried to change the relationship. Perhaps when some time has passed and you have remained firm in your new way of living, they may come to believe that you are different and worthy of their trust. Unfortunately, some people may never be able to trust you again. In AA they call that "the wreckage of our past." As time goes on you will become more at ease with all types of outcomes.

Avoid Self-Destructive Retaliation

It may be very disappointing to you if the person with whom you are trying to reconnect does not want to reopen the relationship or allow it to be healed. You may feel really sad and need to be around people who support you and are on a similar path. This is one of the many times the twelve-step meetings are so helpful. These people have often had similar experiences and may understand better than anyone else how you feel.

But avoid using rejection as an excuse to go back to old behavior. Seeking revenge against someone always has a boomerang effect and only does *you* the harm. Many people have died of alcoholism and drug addiction as a result of drinking or using drugs in retaliation against someone. Others became infected with HIV while they were acting out promiscuously in retaliation against someone.

It is wise never to give anyone that much power over the choices you make. And be careful not to stop working your spiritual program because you are seeking revenge. This is not an easy program to work. It's simple, but it's not easy. But if you choose to do it, you *will* make it through. "This too shall pass," even if it may not feel like it at times.

Be careful not to buckle because of someone's response or lack of response to you. All you can do is pray for the person. Prayers have a remarkable way of working when nothing else can. One of the slogans used in AA is "There, but for the grace of God, go I." If someone rejects you, this slogan may fit the situation. At least today you know that you are trying to heal yourself and your relationships. But not very long ago you may have been the one who refused to accept someone's apology.

Remember that people who are hostile are expressing, through their behavior, their own brokenness. It is their wounded past that cannot give love. No one is born evil or mean. Abused people become abusers because that's all they know. Be careful not to judge the other person or become self-righteous about your newly found spirituality. Thank your Higher Power that you know better now. And keep in mind that "There, but for the grace of God, go I." None of us has a guarantee on how we will act tomorrow.

Making Amends to the Nameless

"What about the nameless? How do I make amends to people if I don't even know who they are or how to find them?" One way is to make a general amends statement or write a general amends letter "to all those persons I hurt when I _____." If you can remember the specific incident it would be even better to write a specific letter, for example, "To the man in Cleveland, I make amends for _____." The writing of the letter, even though you have no place to send it, will offer you a catharsis, a process for releasing the guilt. Then, of course, you must try to not repeat the same behavior.

Making Amends to Those Far Away

"What about the people who are far away?" Telephone calls and letters are best for these people. If you feel you will not be able to say in person or on the telephone what you need to say, a letter may be more appropriate. If you are homosexual or bisexual, you may have left your hometown years ago and not gone back. This is a perfect time to bridge that gap. If the person you call or write to responds positively—which most will—you will be happy to have reconnected with him or her. If you don't hear a positive response, at least you know that you did *your* part. We can't emphasize enough that the phone call or letter should discuss only *your* part in the situation.

Making Amends to the Dead

"What about the people who are dead or for some other reason cannot be contacted?" Owing to the nature of this disease of HIV infection, you may have lost friends and acquaintances to the AIDS virus or you may have unfinished business with a deceased parent or sibling. Therefore, you may have unfinished business with many people who are now dead. This process can be an especially healing one if that is the case.

Write letters to these people. Write each letter as if the person were alive or as if you could give the letter to him or her. Write down exactly what you would like to say in person if you could. You will probably feel a great deal of emotion coming up when you write the letter. You may experience very deep anger and grief. That's okay. It may feel awful, but it is really very healing. Let all of the pent-up feeling out. It's helpful to talk to someone: your counselor, your sponsor, or a friend. You never need be alone again! Always listen to a relaxation tape or do a relaxation exercise after you've completed an emotion-packed letter.

You may wish to visit the cemetery and read the letter aloud at the gravesite or go to a place where you and this person used to go together. The more real and the more active you get in doing this step, the more real and active will be your emotional healing.

Another method is to read the letter to a picture of the person, letting out all of your emotion and probably tears. Making amends with those who have died is a most important step and a very active step. Death does not need to stand in your way.

If you believe in an afterlife, the continuance of life beyond the physical death, imagine yourself talking to the spirit of that person as you look at his or her picture. Remember, this process is for *you;* for *your* emotional release. If you do everything within your power to release your emotion and forgive yourself, you can go on and *not* repeat the same self-defeating behaviors with another person. Unless you make amends to the person, even if he or she is no longer living, you may continue the old behavior pattern, only this time with someone new. That is why we so strongly suggest making *all* amends.

Another way to make amends to persons no longer living is, whenever possible, to be kind and loving to people who are still alive. For example, if the deceased person to whom you wish to make amends is your father, you can be loving to some other older man. You can go out of your way to be helpful while mentally saying, "I'm doing this one for you, Dad." It may sound corny, but it really works.

Financial Amends

We've all heard the saying "Love of money is the root of all evil." Often some of our most inappropriate behavior has been in regard to money. In those cases where you want to make amends concerning a financial issue, be careful to use good judgment. You don't need to jeopardize your own financial security, but you must at least attempt to make restitution by contacting the appropriate persons or institutions and explaining that you are healing.

If you are at all able, it is useful to adopt a restitution schedule, no matter how little you can pay; five dollars a month is better than nothing. If, however, you are in a poor financial situation owing to your illness, it would be foolhardy to risk your health in order to do this. Make a note on your list for amends that you will start restitution when you are able.

SORRY

An interesting article appeared in a San Diego newspaper. It seems that a man awoke one morning to find the driver's car door missing from his new car. The car owner was, naturally, upset and confused. Three years later he received a note, along with six hundred dollars, in the mail. "I am so sorry for taking your car door. I was in a terrible state at that time, and it seemed like a good idea. I am working a program that asks

that I make amends for all the wrongs I have done. Please
accept this money as my attempt to do that. Sincerely, Sorry."
When we read that article we knew "Sorry" was working a
twelve-step program and was on step nine!

Crimes

Similarly, be careful when revealing too much might result in
your losing your job or being jailed, unless you are clear that you
are willing to accept such an outcome. If this is an issue, talk
it over with your sponsor, a good friend, a counselor, or even
an attorney.

Some people have, after careful consideration, actually felt the
need to confess their misdeeds, even when this risked a prison
sentence. Others, after careful consideration, decided it would
harm themselves and their families too much to proceed in this
manner. They chose other means of making amends, such as
writing an anonymous letter to the person harmed, offering an
apology, and resolving never to do it again. They then found other
ways of making fair restitution, such as volunteering in a hospital
or doing civic work. Because they at least addressed the crimes, the
guilt and feelings of not being okay were eased.

Making Amends to Yourself

You may have forgotten that the one person you have probably
harmed the most in your lifetime is yourself. That's true for many
of us. Be gentle and truly make amends to yourself. Try looking
deeply into your eyes in a mirror and telling yourself how sorry
you are for the trouble some of your behavior and ways of thinking
have caused you. It may sound silly at first, but if you hold
eye-to-eye contact with yourself while doing this, a great deal of
emotion may arise. Promise your inner child that you will take
better care of him or her in the future. It's time to be your
own best parent.

Once you have made amends to yourself you will be able to
trust yourself more. Many aspects of this program may seem
simplistic. Let us reassure you that they are not. You make amends

to yourself every time you say no to things that place you in danger. You make amends to yourself every time you treat yourself as a valuable person. Every time you have safe sex, refuse recreational drugs, go to a support group, or talk deeply and honestly with someone, you are making amends to yourself and giving your body messages to live.

Positive Self-Talk: Making Amends

- I choose to accept responsibility for the wreckage of my past.

- I know I can learn to forgive myself and others.

- I can apologize, with full intention to change any behaviors that caused others or myself pain.

- Today my life is full of love and respect. I extend love and respect to others, and they extend the same to me.

- I can accept others' apologies.

- I can allow people who have my highest good in mind back into my life.

- I am given a new chance every time I make amends, a chance to respect and honor myself.

Action Plan for Making Amends

If you did a written fourth-step inventory, you now have a list of people to whom you can make amends. If you did an eighth step, you are probably willing to make some of those amends. The easiest way to do this is to look at your list of names and next to each person's name write down how and when you intend to make your amends.

For people or institutions to whom you can make only partial amends, just make a note next to their names, designating your intent to make amends. Also, indicate how you will make amends to those who are dead or nameless. Your list may look something like this partial list:

Mom—Call tonight. Try to be less judgmental.

Jason—Call tomorrow. Try not to be manipulative.

Dad—Write a letter on his birthday.

Jeffrey—Write a letter next month.

City of San Marcos—Write a letter and send maybe five dollars a month.

Lisa—Talk to today. Spend more quality time with her.

David—Write a letter next week.

Club Fund—Resign as treasurer. Talk to Susan on Wednesday, regarding repayment plan of five dollars a month.

Remember, true amends are not just an apology. They imply a sincere attempt to change the behavior that gave rise to the need for the apology. Words alone are not enough. We need to be willing, like David was, to relate to others in a new way.

Ritual for Making Amends

You can use a ritual to empower yourself before making amends.

Rehearsal

1. Start by centering yourself, relaxing and saying a prayer or affirming to yourself the importance of what you are about to do.

2. Ask your Higher Self, your Higher Power, for guidance and support.

3. Affirm to yourself, I am willing to love and forgive myself and this other person.

4. Bring to mind what you want to say—remember, keep it simple—being certain to speak only of your part in the behavior.

5. Briefly, picture yourself saying this, hear your voice saying

it clearly, and feel your body remaining calm as you do. (A typical amends statement might be "I am involved in a program that suggests that I become aware of the harm I have caused others. I want to take responsibility for my behavior and the ways I have acted. I want to apologize to you for anything I may have done that harmed you in any way [be specific if appropriate]. I promise to be more aware in the future.")

6. Affirm to yourself, I have no expectations of this other person, and am willing to accept however he or she may respond.

7. Imagine that the other person does not respond positively, but you remain just as calm and feel just as whole, concentrating upon a sense of relief. "Well, I did it and I'm so glad it's over."

8. Imagine this person responding as positively as possible, perhaps embracing you and telling you that you are completely forgiven. Allow yourself to accept this.

9. Affirm to yourself, I am now willing to turn this entire matter over to my Higher Power, my Higher Self.

The Real Thing

1. Get in touch with the person in whatever way is appropriate. Do exactly what you have practiced in your imagery.

2. When it is finished, take a little while to relax, perhaps using relaxation tapes or a relaxation process. But first cross the person's name off the list and notice how good that feels.

Ninth-Step Affirmations

Today I choose to start my life over again.

Today I choose to make full amends to myself, as well as others.

Today I reconnect with the people who are important to me.

Today I choose to forgive myself and others.

Today I choose to take better care of my body, my mind, my emotions, and my spirit.

Today I choose to take better care of that precious child who lives inside of me.

Today I am the one responsible for me.

Today I will nurture myself as only I can.

Today I choose to put myself first when it is appropriate.

Today I am assertive and ask for what I need or want.

Today I protect myself from abuse—my own or anyone else's.

TEN

Continuous Self-Appraisal

STEP TEN
CONTINUED **to take** PERSONAL INVENTORY
and when we are WRONG PROMPTLY ADMIT **it.**

CONTINUED *persevered*

PERSONAL *applying to the person, character, or conduct of an individual*

INVENTORY *a list of items, with their worth noted; an evaluation*

WRONG *unsuitable; not what ought to be; incorrect*

PROMPTLY *acting quickly, as occasion demands*

ADMIT *acknowledge; to grant in argument*

Step ten can help you stay on course and avoid accumulating guilt. It can also help keep your relationships flowing freely and harmoniously.

PAUL'S STORY

Paul was not feeling well. When Francis came home, Paul found himself bickering and finding fault with him. An argu-

ment developed and "you always," "you make me," "I really just don't care anymore" came out of both of their mouths. They both said angry things that they did not really mean. Even though Francis said some really awful things too, Paul was able to get himself quiet by going to another room and doing some deep breathing.

Paul asked himself in what way was he at fault. He was able to see that when he was not feeling well he reverted back to his old behavior of finding fault and taking things out on Francis. He was then able to assume responsibility for his part in the event. He went back to Francis and apologized for his behavior, careful not to bring Francis's part into his apology. He was able to say, "Let's start this conversation over. Hi, Francis. How was your day?" They both laughed and felt much better.

Step Ten and HIV Infection

When we are under stress or not feeling well, like Paul we may tend to be irritable and snappish. Often we cause others pain by our remarks. We do not need any additional guilt this pain engenders, and others do not need our unaddressed abuse. To imagine that you will never slip into old behaviors is fantasy. But the tenth step allows you to quickly reconnect with yourself and others and stop further emotional damage.

Staying on Course Through the Tenth Step

Step ten is done on a daily (and sometimes moment-to-moment) basis. It's a maintenance step. In the previous steps you explored your attitudes, feelings, and spiritual connection. Working these steps can help you learn how to accept where you are in life. With that acceptance, a great strength can be born in you, and this strength can help you better deal with the various aspects of your life, including risk of or actual HIV infection or AIDS. Other steps assist in analyzing and gaining a true perspective on how you had been handling life and what you may need to change in order to live life in a more harmonious way, as well as to reconnect you with yourself and others. The tenth step helps ensure that you practice what you have learned in your daily life and that you avoid old patterns that might sap your newfound strength and undermine what acceptance and serenity you've gained.

"But Why Do I Have to Do This Every Day?

One way to keep your life positive and constructive is to make a habit of assessing your emotions, thoughts, and behaviors on a continuous basis. You know your patterns by now. But it takes more than knowledge to change patterns that are deeply ingrained. It is unrealistic to imagine that all of these inappropriate ways of being can be changed overnight.

Thus the tenth step asks for frequent appraisal. Only in this way can you catch yourself quickly when you are not feeling, thinking, or acting in a way that serves you. You can quickly interrupt that particular way of being before it becomes a habit again. But be gentle with yourself. Be your own honest witness, not a judge! Remember, "Easy does it." When you stop any destructive behavior, immediately follow up by forgiving yourself, rather than judging or condemning yourself. Remember, you're aiming for progress here, not perfection!

Permanent positive change, especially in areas that cause damage to your immune system and to your peace of mind, is important for overall health and well-being. Step ten helps you stay honest and humble, while keeping the picture of the person that you are becoming clear in your mind. It allows you to say, "Yes, this is how I *want* to feel, think, and act. This way serves me and others. I am changing the things I need to change. I am becoming more comfortable with who I am and who I am capable of becoming. I am healing. I can do it. I am becoming whole."

Taking the Inventory

We suggest taking an inventory, assessing yourself, at least once a day. You may need to stop right in the middle of the day and do an inventory. The minute you feel uncomfortable, stop and find out what is going on. It's a spiritual axiom that whenever we feel uncomfortable there is something wrong with the way we are thinking or acting. Ask yourself, What am I doing? Why am I uncomfortable? Are you putting up with abuse? Are you allowing an incident in the present to pull you into the past and feeling overwhelmed by old resentments? It's important to really live one day (perhaps one second) at a time.

Finding Yourself in Fear

"What should I do if I'm afraid?" Fear is a natural, normal emotion designed to warn us that something we value is in danger. But staying in the fear as a helpless victim is self-defeating. Let the fear motivate you to do something positive with it. Take an inventory of the fear. Ask the fear what it is trying to tell you. Is the fear telling you that you are not living in the present? Remind yourself that today is today, and next week is next week; we all get lost in projection, but now you're aware and can choose to do something different.

Or is the fear telling you that you are not doing what you know you could be doing? Are you fearful because you have not been using safe sex and have been placing yourself and others in jeopardy? Have you been drinking alcohol or using recreational drugs? Have you been eating correctly and resting enough? Have you been following the suggestions of your health care professionals? Have you been assertive about your needs? Have you been sharing your feelings with others? Have you been doing your affirmations and relaxation exercises?

Let the fear talk to you and tell you what it is all about. Feel the fear but don't just stay in it! Do something with it. Sitting in the fear only makes stress chemicals, which can suppress your immune system further.

Or is the fear telling you that you are in regret, resentment, guilt, anger? What can you do about these feelings? These all come from the past. What can you do about the past? Is there any unfinished business hanging around? You may wish to consult your list from step eight. Is there someone on that list to whom you still need to make amends?

Or have you recently done something about which you feel badly? Is there anything you can do about it? If there is, then *do it*. You can call that person or write that letter; make amends in any way that is appropriate. You can pray for forgiveness if forgiveness is needed: forgiveness of yourself or forgiveness of others. Working with others also helps. Are you afraid because you have some unfinished business regarding legal or death-related matters? Read Chapter 13 and take care of whatever matter is bothering you. But try to get back into the present moment and do something that can stop the anxiety.

Sometimes we get afraid and simply can't figure out why. This feeling is often described as a pervading sense of impending doom. We're just plain afraid. But "just being afraid" is still a very uncomfortable, sometimes even paralyzing, feeling. Please call someone. Someone needs to hear from you. Someone needs to know that when he or she is afraid, he or she can use your example and reach out for help too.

Don't "Should" Me: Expectations

Or are you uncomfortable because you have unmet expectations of yourself or others? Unfortunately, the more expectations you have, the less chance you have to find peace. Remember the Serenity Prayer; the only thing you can change is yourself.

Placing expectations on others is one way we set ourselves up for unhappiness. Do you keep expecting people to change to be the way you would like them to be? Do you keep going to people, expecting to get something that they are incapable of giving or unwilling to give? Do you, metaphorically, keep going to the hardware store to buy milk, even though you *know* it doesn't carry it?

We are all much more comfortable when we lower our expectations. Try changing your shoulds to coulds. It's amazing how different that feels. Try changing your expectations to preferences. Listen to the difference: "I expect you to change." "I prefer it if you change." As we said before, it is very important for your overall health that you have healthy relationships, and this attitude can help ensure that.

Examine your beliefs and assumptions carefully. Perhaps you don't state your needs clearly, instead assuming that the other person knows what you need or want. Being self-responsible includes clearly stating your needs. Then the other person can choose whether to satisfy them. When you keep your needs unspoken you only set up the "martyr game," which guarantees resentment on your part and the part of others. Sometimes you might expect others to meet needs that they don't even know you have! This is just another example of codependency: giving your power away to others. Unspoken needs become unmet needs, and unmet needs build resentment. Resentment, in turn, poisons your mind, your body, and your relationships. Most unhappiness in relationships comes from unmet expectations, and expectations are most often unmet because they are unknown.

Remember, only *you* can take care of your emotional needs. If you clearly let your needs be known and yet keep turning to someone who is unable to meet them, accept that person's limitations and get your needs met in another way. Many people spend a lifetime waiting for spouses or parents to understand them. And, sad as it is, sometimes they just never do. Though it may be difficult, accepting that fact will create more contentment in the long run than continuing to wish that they would. Stop going to the hardware store for milk. You're never going to find it there!

Accept Where You Find Yourself

One of the purposes of this inventory is to accept negative feelings when they come up, and explore them. Therein lies the power of the inventory. Some people live their lives in anger, denying they are angry and never giving themselves a chance to explore the anger. Before embarking on an investigation, however, we all need to accept our humanness. No human being is perfect. Humans do things that they need to stop doing. It is part of the human condition. So please do yourself a big favor and drop any perfectionism, so that you can accept where you are and do something about it.

Refer to Chapter 2, for the lists of ways of thinking that set you up for failure. This will clarify for you what is really behind your anger and other emotions. Most mind traps and other often unconscious ways of responding are clearly explained there. When you find yourself placing too many demands on yourself or others, or being too aggressive or submissive, these lists can help you regain clarity.

Soon this will be a snap. When you feel yourself becoming uncomfortable, you will be able to recognize that you are either in the past or the future, or placing too many expectations on others, or responding out of some misbelief from childhood. You will find yourself saying, "Uh-oh, another expectation crept in on me." Or, "Oh, I'm in the past or the future again. I need to get back into the present. Okay, what am I doing right now? Where am I? I'm driving the car. Good, then I will drive the car!" "But I can't get that out of my mind! What can I do? Oh, I know, I can put on my affirmation tape and listen to it." Or, "I'll yell at the telephone poles or sing or swear loudly and then go home and take a shower and wash these thoughts and feelings right down the drain."

There are solutions. There are things you can do. It's up to you to choose a solution and then carry it out.

"When We Are Wrong Promptly Admit It"

When you find yourself doing something you don't feel good about, something that keeps you from being loving and respectful, the tenth step asks you to *promptly* admit your error. Paul took some time out until he could get a handle on why he was being nasty to Francis, and then he returned to apologize. You too need to let others know that you don't want to do anything that will cause them to withdraw from you. You probably don't mean to withhold your Higher Self from them. We all know how we'd like to act, but none of us is a saint. We all snap, yell, and respond with knee-jerk reactions that can push away the people to whom we want to be closest.

You can apologize and promise yourself and them to avoid repeating the same mistake. You might say something like this: "I'm sorry. I want you to know that when I act like that I really don't mean it. It doesn't fit with how I feel about you, and I'm trying to change. Soon I hope my actions will fit more closely with how I feel about you." Afterward you will sense a freedom: freedom from the self-contempt and guilt that you carry around when you are not meeting your own standards. This statement also frees you to reconnect with another immediately, before any more damage to your relationship occurs.

There may be certain individuals whom you simply don't like. If you try to keep justice and courtesy as your key motives you will find that you can deal with these people more easily. Remember that there are still other people who remain emotionally ill or are frequently wrong. "There, but for the grace of God, go I": it would serve no purpose to get into an angry encounter or arguing match. Remember, this is *your* life, *your* program of recovery, and *your* peace of mind is the goal. Fruitless debates only waste your time and energy.

Making It Easier on Yourself

Try to spend most of your time with people who uplift and inspire you, not those who drag you down. You are easily influenced by the company you keep. If you are frequently in the company of people who are negative, complaining, or behaving in ways that are inappropriate and harmful, it is difficult to rise above that kind of influence. The kind of people you need to be surrounded and supported by are those who have taken responsibility for their lives, who are aspiring to do better.

The company you keep is food for your spirit. It is every bit as important as the medicine you take or the water you drink. You would not want to make your body sick by drinking contaminated water. Likewise, you don't want to contaminate your spirit with foul companions.

Ending Your Day

Before going to sleep each night, most people who follow a twelve-step program do a tenth step regarding their day. You do that by picturing all the things you did that you feel good about and thanking your Higher Power or Higher Self, for helping you be true to your Higher Nature. Also picture briefly the things you want to do differently, using the script from step seven—"Image Rehearsal for a New Inner Script." In your mind's eye practice how you want to do things the next time. Let your mind take in that picture on a deep level.

As you are going to sleep, repeat some loving affirmations on your own. If an event scheduled for the next day worries you, imagine it going well and then verbally affirm over and over as you drift off to sleep a positive affirmation, such as, "I'm calm and serene. I have a loving heart."

You might want to relax now using a relaxation tape or the loving light exercise in Chapter 1, or the spiritual attunement exercise in Chapter 2.

Tenth-Step Affirmations

Today I choose to keep my power by assuming responsibility for my thoughts, words, and deeds.

Today I remain alert for any resentment or dishonesty on my part and deal with it immediately.

Today I look at my motives and steer clear of manipulation and attempting to please others at my own expense.

Today I am fully responsible for myself.

Today when I am wrong I promptly admit it.

Today I choose to acknowledge the positive aspects of my nature as well as the negative.

Today I use my mistakes as a map for how I choose to *not* act next time.

ELEVEN

Daily Prayer and Meditation

STEP ELEVEN
SOUGHT through PRAYER and MEDITATION
to IMPROVE our CONSCIOUS CONTACT with God
as we understand God, praying only for
KNOWLEDGE of God's WILL for us, and
the POWER TO CARRY THAT OUT

SOUGHT *went in search of; took pains to find*

PRAYER *a solemn petition for help addressed to the Higher Power*

MEDITATION *close or continued thought*

IMPROVE *to make better; to increase the good qualities*

CONSCIOUS *having direct knowledge of a thing; aware*

CONTACT *a state of touching or connection*

KNOWLEDGE *the clear and certain perception of truth and fact*

WILL *wish; desire*

POWER *ability; strength; energy manifested in action*

TO CARRY THAT OUT *to sustain to the end*

Step eleven gives you the tools to continuously deepen your spiritual connection, which brings you the serenity you seek and deserve. You can learn how meditation and prayer not only help your mind and emotions, but also assist you in your physical healing.

ALEX'S STORY

Since Alex has been working a twelve-step program his days from dawn to dusk are quite different. He is now usually able to awaken to the music of his clock radio rather than having to use the blaring alarm. He starts his day by saying his affirmations, and while showering does his healing imagery. Alex focuses his attention on the water and his body, so that he really feels the water as it flows down over him. He imagines the shower water to be a soothing light totally covering him, bringing him healing and protection, from the top of his head to the tips of his toes. He imagines the white light extending from above the top of his head to under the bottoms of his feet, to the right of him and to the left of him, in front of him and behind him. He feels warm and protected, totally enclosed in a sphere of healing light. Some days as he dresses he listens to his affirmation tape and thanks his body for working for him.

As Alex sits in front of his window breathing deeply, or while eating breakfast, he reads from his daily meditation book. He relaxes and meditates for a few minutes on what he has read or uses his favorite mantra, which is, "I give only love; I receive only love." He affirms in his mind that he is cared for by his Higher Power and asks for guidance in his new day. He asks to be of service to himself and others and tells his Higher Power that he surrenders his will to him.

While driving to work Alex listens to a pleasant tape rather than playing the radio roulette game. He chooses to be aware enough to avoid wasting his energy on petty annoyances that he cannot control—"Accept the things I cannot change"—such as the traffic. He tries to transform any negative experiences by staying alert to any possible good that can come out of irritating or painful events. If he gets stuck in traffic, he smiles and says to his Higher Power, "Cute, another opportunity to develop tolerance. Just what I needed! Well, I guess the worst thing that can happen is I will be late. I've been late before and have lived through it. I don't think it will kill me this time. Maybe I should start getting up earlier."

Today Alex chooses to be more aware of his body. He eats carefully and takes his vitamins and medication. He also stays tuned in to how much rest his body needs and takes breaks as often as possible. He no longer chooses to fill his mind with negative chatter, so while he's eating in the morning and in the evening, he leaves the news off and reads an inspirational story or a book of cartoons.

Throughout his day when Alex feels upset, overwhelmed, or anxious, he usually remembers to stop and take some deep breaths, imagining his healing light filling his body, starting at this feet, and asks for guidance from his Higher Power.

When he's in bed Alex reflects on his day. He brings to mind the positive occurrences and thanks his Higher Power. He also recalls reactions of his that he would like to change the next time similar circumstances occur. Alex is very aware that his mind can't take a joke, and so he is careful to quickly let go of negative thoughts and replace them with positive ones. Rather than beat himself up for what he did that he wished he hadn't, he holds the image in his mind of how he wants to respond the next time. In this way his mind can take in the positive impression. Alex knows that he can do things differently now if he chooses, and that by reprogramming his mind with the outcome he wants, he is making the achievement of that outcome easier. He listens to his affirmation tape or repeats one of his favorite affirmations—"I am a child of God and my Father loves me" or "I have exactly what I need when I need it"—and finds a peaceful sea of calm slowing his brain and lulling him to sleep.

Step Eleven and HIV Infection

Step three said that we decided to "turn our wills and our lives over to the care of God as we understand God," step five that we "admitted to the God of our understanding, to ourselves and to another human being the exact nature of our wrongs," and step seven that we "humbly asked the God of our understanding to remove our shortcomings." So if you are using the steps you have been communicating with your Higher Power throughout the entire program. The eleventh step allows you to deepen that contact, and let it permeate your entire existence. It frees up your energy to be used for your healing and comforts you when you feel needy.

A relationship with God, your Higher Power as you understand that, is like any other relationship: it requires nurturing and attention. Emotional involvement and repetition are the keys to developing and maintaining any behavior. This is also true of your contact with your Higher Power. Step eleven is one way to work on your relationship with your Higher Power.

How to Pray

The concept of prayer may be familiar to you, but perhaps maintaining it on a daily basis is not. Or perhaps, owing to some experience in the past, you have had a difficult time relating to a Higher Power. If you worked on step three you have by now developed some concept of God, a Higher Power, or a Higher Self. If you have not developed such a concept you might want to reread chapters 2 and 3. Step eleven not only asks that we pray, but also suggests that we pray "for knowledge of God's will for us, and the power to carry that out." As you probably realized in step three, your Higher Power, or Higher Self, knows much better what is in your best interest than your ego-directed mind does. Remember that your mind has been conditioned by your past experiences to "think" it knows what is best for you, but this is not always the case. How many times have you prayed or wished for something, and, when you got it, found that it was not what you really needed or wanted?

As you saw in step three, it is your Higher Self, who works from your heart, who really knows what is best for you. Your Higher Self has no ego to filter through, and therefore does not send out warped messages, as your mind can. This is the reason it is suggested that you do not pray for specific things. The things you want may not be what is truly best for you. The principles of a twelve-step program suggest that instead we pray for our Higher Power's will to make itself known and then for the power to carry that out.

The method used when praying can be as individual as the person. Some people pray with formal prayers; others talk as if in conversation. Some people have a set time they pray and others pray on and off all day. Some pray on their knees next to their beds, some while lying in their beds, others while in the shower, driving their cars, or taking walks. How, when, and where you pray is up to you. Your relationship with your Higher Power is a very personal one. We don't feel a need to emphasize the logistics of prayer, only its role.

GAIL'S STORY

Gail wanted to have a relationship with Robin from almost the minute she first noticed him. She was sure that it was her Higher Power's will; after all, she had met him at a meeting and heard him share so easily how he felt. He seemed to have a solid spiritual base and they had so much in common: a match made in heaven. She was sure he was "the one" and prayed nightly for him to notice her. Sure enough, he did, and they began a relationship. Gail moved in to his apartment, and within two weeks she discovered he was not the person she had thought he was. She had an awful time trying to discuss anything with Robin or trying to come to any compromise with him about anything.

Every time Gail threatened to break up with him or move out, Robin assured her that he would change and things would be different if she would only give him another chance. He said that he could not live without her, would have nothing left to live for without her. He turned words around so fast she wasn't sure what he was saying, and she felt so confused she thought one of them was crazy. She couldn't understand how he could be so charming and sweet one minute, and hostile and sarcastic the next.

It took a long time before Gail could get up enough courage to end the relationship. Her counselor told her that Robin was a master manipulator, but many people thought Robin was well balanced and charismatic, and Gail often felt confused about how she felt and what to do. Finally she came to know that it didn't matter what people thought. She was the one in the situation and if she knew it was not healthy, then it was up to her to do something about it. But she was really afraid that Robin would try to kill himself, and she didn't want to feel responsible.

After some counseling she came to know that she did not have power over Robin's life, and that if Robin lost the will to live or was going to kill himself there was nothing she could do. Her responsibility was to end the relationship as kindly and honestly as possible. It was a hard lesson to learn, but now Gail prays only to know the will of her Higher Power. She understands that people and things are not always as they seem. She does not always know what is truly in her best interests, but her Higher Power does.

"The Power to Carry that Out"

"The power to carry that out" means exactly what it says. For example, you know it is best to engage in only safe sex, abstain from drugs and alcohol, and avoid negative self-talk. But these may be very old patterns you are trying to break, and you may find it very difficult. That is why you need to always ask for the power to do what you know is the will of your Higher Power. Very often it is much easier to do *your* will and stay stuck in your old self-defeating behaviors, even when you know they are definitely not your Higher Power's will. Just because something is good for you does *not* mean it is the easier way! The way of least resistance is always the way of old habit patterns. That's why we suggest staying linked to your Higher Power through prayer and meditation. This will give you the power to carry out what you know in your heart is best for you.

Daily Third Step

When you completed step three you turned your will and your life over to the care of God as you understand God. You may ask, So why do I have to do this each and every day? Because it is very easy to forget the resolves of yesterday. (Remember the slogan "One day at a time.") That is why it is important to rededicate yourself each and every day. As imperfect human beings, we tend to slip back into old self-defeating ways of being when things get rough. Therefore we suggest that you start your day off with the third-step prayer in Chapter 3, and throughout the day repeat to yourself, "Not my will, Lord, but thine be done" or "Thy will be done."

Or you could talk to your Higher Power like you would a good friend. There were times when all Gail could say was, "Reporting in for duty: act, speak, and think for me today. I really don't feel very good or very spiritual right now, but I know somehow you and I can handle it! Thanks!"

How to Meditate

Study after study has demonstrated the benefits of meditation for not only mental and emotional illnesses, but also physical ones. Dr. Janice Kiecolt-Glaser observed that elderly persons who meditated were able to improve the function of their immune systems, evidenced not only in laboratory test results, but also in the reduction of upper respiratory tract infections. Another study, using an experienced meditator, demonstrated that she was able to change how her body responded to an injection of chicken pox virus. When she meditated and focused on her arm not reacting, the reaction was much less than when she did not! Other studies have shown that during meditation heart rate and breathing slows, oxygen consumption is lowered, and less lactic acid is produced (which means the body is using energy more efficiently). Dr. Herbert Benson referred to this unique state brought on by meditation as the "relaxation response," which recharges the human body and mind and facilitates healing; it is the opposite of the stress response. The importance of this finding is obvious for anyone infected with HIV.

Prayer and meditation feed the mind and spirt like food and oxygen feed the body. We all need physical, emotional, and spiritual support. One way you can find it is in daily prayer and meditation. This is the foundation on which a happy and serene life can be built.

Prayer is often referred to as talking to God; meditation is referred to as listening to God. The relaxation exercises in this program are a type of meditation. Many people find that looking at a wonder of nature, such as the calm of the ocean, a flower in bloom, a bird in flight, or even a piece of fruit or a blade of grass, can be inspiring and comforting. Additionally, you may choose a prayer-based meditation, where you read a poem or prayer and reflect on it quietly. Many use the Lord's Prayer; others are fond of the prayer of St. Francis of Assisi or the Universal Prayer.

We have included the last two prayers here for you. You may wish to copy them onto index cards and post them on the dashboard of your car or on your bathroom mirror to help you keep your perspective.

THE PRAYER OF SAINT FRANCIS OF ASSISI

Lord, make me an instrument of Thy peace.
Where there is hatred, let me sow love;
Where there is injury, pardon;
Where there is doubt, faith;
Where there is despair, hope;
Where there is darkness, light;
And where there is sadness, joy.
Divine Master, grant that I may not so much seek to be
    consoled as to console;
To be understood as to understand;
To be loved as to love.
For it is in giving that I receive,
It is in pardoning that I am pardoned,
And it is in dying that I am born to eternal life!

THE UNIVERSAL PRAYER

Eternal Reality, You are Everywhere.
You are Infinite Unity, Truth and Love;
You permeate our souls,
Every corner of the Universe, and beyond.

To some of us You are Father, Friend or Partner, to others,
Higher Power, Higher Self or Inner Self.
To many of us, You are all these and more.
You are within us and we within You.
We know You forgive our trespasses if we forgive ourselves
and others.
We know You protect us from destructive temptation if
we continue to seek Your help and guidance.
We know You provide us food and shelter today if we but
place our trust in You and try to do our best.
Give us this day knowledge of Your will for us and the
power to carry it out.
For Yours is Infinite Power and Love, Forever. Amen

Just let the words bathe your heart while your mind is silent. You may hear a quiet little voice speak to you either during your meditation or sometime during the day. If you hear something comforting and loving, know that it is your Higher Power, or Higher Self, talking to you. If it says anything other than loving, know that it is just your ego rebelling, probably quoting some old tape of the past. We suggest that you thank it for sharing its thoughts and immediately dismiss it; don't even argue with it. Just let it go.

Some people choose to use a mantra, which is just a word or phrase quietly repeated over and over with each breath. Repeating *I am* on inhalation and words such as *love, peace, forgiving, accepting, calm,* or *relaxed* on exhalation is one way of using a mantra. Others prefer saying their first names on inhalation and phrases such as *let go* or *stay calm* on exhalation. You may choose to use a word with special religious meaning, such as *Jesus, God, Master,* or *shalom.* Whatever short word or phrase is soothing and brings you peace will work.

Meditation not only helps to calm you emotionally, but also relaxes you physically. It helps to release the negative energy accumulated during the many stresses of the day. Once released, this energy becomes available to you for constructive pursuits, and can refresh and uplift your state of mind. Studies on people who meditate repeatedly demonstrate increased memory, better concentration, and an overall increased feeling of well-being.

It's best to start off with just a few minutes each day and slowly increase the time. Make sure you are in a quiet place where you won't be disturbed. Unplug the phone, get into a comfortable position, and use a blanket if you tend to become chilled. If distracting thoughts come into your mind, just let them go, like a passing breeze. You do not need to fight the distracting thoughts or judge them or yourself. Everyone has this problem in the beginning, and even after years of meditating, outside thoughts still come. Just refocus on your mantra or your meditation thought. Because we all have such busy minds, at first it is much easier to use a tape of soft music or one of a gentle voice that guides you through meditation. Once you become used to being quiet for twenty minutes with the tape you will find it much easier to be quiet without the assistance of a tape. It will become easier with practice—we promise!

Throughout Your Day

Even when you start your day off with prayer and meditation, sometimes the events of the day can be discouraging. If you find yourself upset or uncomfortable, you might quietly say to yourself some comforting phrase, slogan, or prayer. "Make me an instrument of thy peace," "Easy does it," "Turn it over," or The Serenity Prayer are frequently helpful. Any phrase or words that will reconnect you with your Higher Self, or Higher Power, will give you great comfort, peace, and clarity of mind.

The "Big Book" of AA (page 87) says it like this: "As we go through the day we pause, when agitated or doubtful, and ask for the right thought or action. We constantly remind ourselves that we are no longer running the show, humbly saying to ourselves many times each day 'Thy will be done.' We are then in much less danger of excitement, fear, anger, worry, self-pity, or foolish decisions. We become much more efficient. We do not tire so easily, for we are not burning up energy foolishly as we did when we were trying to arrange life to suit ourselves." Those of us who have used this method can tell you that it is not just magical thinking: it really works.

Also remember that you have choices today. Just because your shoelace broke first thing in the morning and you ran out of gas and spilled your juice, or even if something much more serious or frustrating happened, it does not mean that you have to have an awful day. Even if you forgot to pray and turn your will and life over to your Higher Power, it's never too late. You can restart your day anytime you want. Just say to yourself, "That's it, I'm starting this day over! Okay, Higher Power, you may have noticed that this day has not been going very well. I could use some assistance about now. I'm starting this day over!"

Putting Your Day to Rest

Before going to sleep, again try quieting yourself in prayer and meditation. Use any of the prayers already mentioned or any other of your choosing. Remember that what goes in your mind is very important to your mental health.

Listening to heavy rock music, or watching the news or a violent television show is not what your mind needs, especially right before going to bed. If you want peaceful sleep, read or listen to something that is inspiring and comforting before you end your day. Listening to soft music or reading a religious or spiritual book or poem is a good way to relax your mind and body before sleep.

If you made or purchased an affirmation tape it's useful to listen to it during the day, but it is especially helpful to also listen to it right before or while falling asleep. Remember, put into your mind what you want to come out. Garbage in, garbage out. Inspiration, affirmation in; inspiration, affirmation out.

This principle is especially important when you are waking up or falling asleep. This is when your brain has alpha and theta brain waves, so your mind is very programmable. Be careful what you program! Because the brain is so programmable at this time, many people use affirmations right before sleep and immediately upon arising. Two of our own favorites are "I'm a child of God and my Father loves me" and "I have exactly what I need when I need it."

Eleventh-Step Affirmations

Today I choose to improve my conscious contact with my Higher Power.

Today I choose to start off my day by asking my Higher Power for guidance and courage.

Today I choose to stop often and silently repeat my favorite phrase or prayer, which helps me stay centered.

Today if I become upset or anxious I choose to stop and ask my Higher Power for direction.

Today at the end of the day I choose to reflect and give thanks to my Higher Power.

Today I choose to allow prayer and meditation to nurture me.

TWELVE

Working with Others And Sharing Ourselves

STEP TWELVE

Having had a SPIRITUAL AWAKENING as the RESULT of these steps, we tried TO CARRY this MESSAGE to other persons at risk or infected with HIV, and PRACTICE these PRINCIPLES in all our AFFAIRS

SPIRITUAL *not material; holy; divine*

AWAKENING *arousal from a state resembling sleep; new life*

RESULT *consequence; outcome; effect*

TO CARRY *to act as a bearer; to lead or urge in a moral sense*

MESSAGE *any communication, written or verbal, sent from one person to another*

PRACTICE *to do frequently or habitually; to do*

PRINCIPLES *governing laws of conduct; settled rules of action*

AFFAIRS *matters; concerns; business of any kind*

Step twelve can help reinforce your spiritual principles while you help those who still suffer.

Step Twelve and HIV Infection

Part of being spiritually awake is to feel love and compassion for other human beings. The desire to share that awakened state is a natural outcome of knowing the pain of living under the cloud of any crisis, such as HIV infection. The twelfth step encourages that sharing and interaction with others. Developing the ability to express this spiritually awakened state in thought, word, and deed is a lifelong process. This ability is sharpened with each connection with another person that you make. It is in "giving it away" that you keep your spirit alive and well. The twelfth step assures you that whether you are at risk of developing HIV or are already infected, you can be of service to others in a way that is life enhancing for you, as well as for them.

Remember, this is a process that occurs over time. We encourage you to proceed at your own pace. If you do not yet feel ready to actively help others, please be gentle with yourself. There are many other ways to help people, as we will discuss. In the meantime, just by taking care of yourself you serve as a good example to others. Being true to yourself is always the most important thing you can do, and setting a good example is very important. Know that at some time you may feel ready to be more actively involved. If that time is not now, that is okay. When the time is right you will know it.

> The only ones among you who will be really happy
> are those who will have sought and found how to serve.
> —Albert Schweitzer, M.D.

MARY'S STORY

Mary is a middle-aged schoolteacher who became infected with HIV through a blood transfusion. She has always been a bright ray of sunshine in the life of everyone who knows her. AIDS has not stopped that. But she has needed to make many transformations in her thinking to accommodate a life-threatening disease and still remain optimistic. Being a teacher, Mary understands how important role models can be. Therefore she works with others, offering her experience, strength, and hope on a regular basis.

Over the years she has done a variety of things that are consistent with the twelfth step. On occasion she becomes politically involved and spends time obtaining funding and getting laws changed. She speaks at conferences and visits with politicians. Other times she quietly lends a supportive ear to someone who has been newly diagnosed with AIDS. She remains very aware of how important her connection with others is to her own sense of well-being. There are also times when she feels tired and honors that by pulling in the reins and canceling engagements. At such times she often uses the telephone as her link to the outside world.

Mary feels that one of her reasons for living is to be available to learn from, as well as teach, others that which she has learned. Keeping the slogan in mind, "First things first," she is able to balance her time and energy so that she doesn't exhaust herself or give too much of herself away. Because of that kind of thinking, even when she needs to pull back from commitments she is aware that she serves as a good example of how one needs to respect one's own limitations.

As you can tell, Mary is working intensely on her twelfth step. In so doing she gives and receives the kind of love and friendship that make life worth living. Her struggle is not easy, but clearly she feels it is worth it!

"Having Had a Spiritual Awakening"

There are as many varieties of spiritual awakening as there are people. Some will experience it gradually; for others it will come suddenly. The essence of the awakening is, however, the knowledge that you are no longer alone in this struggle called life. The distinguished American psychologist William James, in his book *Varieties of Religious Experience*, indicates a multitude of ways in which people have discovered their spirituality.

One of the characteristics of long-term survivors of a life-threatening illness is that they are able to find new meaning as a result of their illness, and a sense of purpose in their lives. Like them, you may be beginning to understand the value of having a new level of awareness of your being. Life is not a dead end, something to be endured. You can discover your own inner strength, an inner knowing that there is more to life than you perhaps had previously known. You now probably possess more honesty, tolerance, peace of mind, love, and selflessness, viewing each day as a gift and each "problem" as a lesson or challenge. Allowing your Higher Power, your Higher Self, to do for you that which you are unable to do for yourself makes life so much simpler.

Review of the Twelve Steps and HIV Infection

If you have been using the twelve steps you may have found that the first step allows you to face the awesome paradox that by accepting and surrendering to the truth of risk of, or actual infection with HIV, you can then go on to do something positive about the way in which your body, mind, and spirit respond to this truth. Like other long-term survivors, you can accept the reality of the diagnosis, yet refuse to view the condition as a death sentence. In claiming powerlessness over HIV you become powerful over yourself!

Step two can lead you to become aware of the ways in which you think and react that fail to serve you. Through its message you can learn to allow your Higher Power to restore you to sane thinking and thus avoid undue stress. The third step helps you turn your will and your life over to your Higher Power, to drop the heavy burden HIV has brought to your life.

Step four's inventory leads you through an honest inventory of yourself and your life. Step five suggests that you share this inventory, in this way reconnecting with yourself. The sixth step recommends you become willing to release any character flaws you found in working step four, so that in the seventh step you can surrender these defects to your Higher Power and ask that power to work in your life to remove them, thus healing you.

Step eight helps you look at how your behavior may have damaged relationships in your life; step nine gives you a model for repairing these disharmonies and recommitting yourself to relationships in a healthier manner.

Step ten shows you how reassessing yourself on a continuous basis is the foundation for avoiding undue guilt and separation from yourself and others. Step eleven gives you a way to maintain and deepen a relationship with your Higher Power. All of these steps can be tools for a happy, joyous, and free life.

So Now What?

Now, like Mary, you may want to carry the message of hope and serenity you have found as a result of this type of thinking and acting. Another characteristic of certain long-term survivors is that they are altruistically involved with others. You probably know many people who are suffering and could use a gentle, hopeful message and a warm smile. Other people who are at risk of infection or infected need what you have gained from this philosophy. They need the support of someone who has already been there. No matter what calamity befalls us in life, the load always seems lighter when we share it with someone who has actually experienced the same tragedy. This is the basic philosophy of the AA fellowship: one alcoholic helping another. It has saved millions of otherwise hopeless individuals.

You are in a unique position to be of service to others in a way that someone who is not infected or at risk of infection could never be. And you now have new tools and a new perspective on what you once probably considered the worst thing that had ever happened to you. By sharing these tools with others, you can make a real difference in their lives and your own. More than likely you will gain as much, if not more than, the person you are helping.

Keeping It by Giving It Away

In using the twelve-step principles in your daily life you are not only modeling for others but also reinforcing your own beliefs. Every time you share the attitudes you have learned with another person, you deepen your own knowing. Every time you listen to another, you are deepening your own healing.

This sharing is also another way of giving your body the

message that you want to live. By actively living each day you say to your immune system, "I'm busy. I have a purpose. I have things to do, so please keep me healthy so I can get on with it!" Your body senses your commitment to life and likewise commits itself.

In stepping out of your own experience you can benefit in many ways. It is easy to get so caught up in what is going on in your own life that you start to feel sorry for yourself. This can lead to prolonged depression and anxiety, which are dangerous to your immune system. The best way to "get out of yourself" is to work with others. Suddenly your problems will seem to fade, and the action you are taking in helping another human being will make you feel much better about yourself. You can have a purpose, a new meaning in life. Only you are in a position to turn this tragedy into a wonderful gift!

The act of giving energizes the giver. History shows that the people who are the happiest are those who dedicate themselves to the service of others. Look at Mother Teresa, Dr. Tom Dooley, Martin Luther King, Jr., Mahatma Gandhi. Remember the joy of giving gifts at Christmas and on birthdays? Who got the more joy out of that: the giver or the receiver?

So How Do I Do This?

You learn to give by practicing the twelve-step principles in all your affairs. That means setting a good example. In following a twelve-step program you are reborn. People may notice and comment on how you've changed. If you wish, you can respond by telling them about twelve-step programs. That person may want to investigate further. You could refer him or her to this book or any twelve-step program that seems appropriate. You may want to offer to help the person with the steps, that is, to be his or her sponsor. This time *you* can be there for someone else, perhaps even listening to his or her fifth step.

Or you may not be doing the steps per se, but rather using the imagery, twelve-step slogans, and twelve-step philosophy in a general manner. You may want to become involved politically, personally act as someone's buddy or helper, work an information or crisis phone line, or do behind-the-scenes clerical work. You can be as close to or as far from people who are sick as you wish. There are many, many ways to help; one of them can fit your talents, situation, preference, and energy level.

You need not do anything big or dramatic to be of service; it's the little things in life that matter and there are probably many little things that you can do. You can help in any way that you are capable, such as cooking, writing letters, driving, sharing at meetings, or talking on the phone. You know how lonely those in your situation can be. You can be there for someone! You can share yourself, share your story. There is always *something* you can do and *someone* who needs the help!

This disease has affected every nation and every type of person on this planet. There are infected babies who are well enough to go home but who live out their short lives in hospitals because their mothers don't want them or are too ill to take care of them. They could certainly use someone to visit and rock them. There are little boys with hemophilia who are shunned by their friends, and mothers who have sold their homes and left their jobs to take care of their sick sons. In certain cities 50 percent of the population of gay and bisexual men and IV drug users are infected. Depending on the type and severity of hemophilia, between 32 and 92 percent of hemophiliacs have been infected. Fear and anger immobilizes these families. You may be in one of these categories. *You* need support; *all these people* need support. We get that which we give. You could offer to stay with a sick person while his or her main support person gets a rest, or do some errands to make his or her life easier. You could take a boy to a baseball game, accompany a friend on a walk in the park, or stuff envelopes. But taking the action—getting out of yourself and helping someone—is the spirit of the twelfth step!

Be careful, however, not to expose yourself to people who continue in self-destructive behaviors. If you engaged in such behaviors in the past, you need to keep in mind that your newfound way of being may still be fragile, and you don't want to risk your own health. Remember that it is not your job to change anyone or seek anyone else's approval, but simply to share your story and your feelings. Also, try not to get too invested in getting anyone else well: not everyone may want to change or be ready to heal at all levels. But, if your friends continue to choose to kill themselves through their behavior, you can let them do it without your having to watch. Remember, just do the footwork; leave the results up to them and their Higher Power.

Social Support Research

We cannot stress enough the importance of getting into some kind of support group, as well as working with others! Many studies have been done on the effect of social support and health, both in animals and humans. These relationships help buffer harmful health effects from psychosocial stress and other hazards.

A large study, one that looked at almost five thousand adults in Alameda County, California, examined the social network index of these individuals and followed them over nine years. The social network included marriage, contacts with extended family and friends, church membership, and formal and informal group affiliations. The study took into account such factors as physical health, smoking, and obesity. They found that people low on the index, meaning those with few social interactions, were *twice* as likely to die as people high on the index.

A similar study, one in Tecumseh, Michigan, looked at almost three thousand adults between ages thirty-five and sixty-nine. The group was followed for ten to twelve years. Controlling for age, blood pressure, and many other significant factors, they found the men with few social ties were *two to three times* more likely to die than the men with many social ties, and the women with little social support were *one and a half to two times* as likely to die than their counterparts with a lot of social support.

Many studies are producing the same kind of data. We know that we are social beings and that isolation causes disease, even death. This information is especially important in dealing with this disease of HIV infection and the feelings of alienation and fear it causes. Many people are still ignorant of the methods of transmission; those who are infected know quite well how these misperceptions can destroy your social relationships.

These kinds of feelings can lead to isolation and depression if you do not take an active stand in fighting against them. The public is becoming more informed and less prejudiced, but it is still not safe to openly discuss your HIV infection in many areas. Unfortunately, this is not the kind of illness you can freely discuss at most workplaces and receive sympathy. Therefore it is even more important for anyone infected with HIV to search out and become involved with groups that render support in this illness. Every moderate-sized town now has an AIDS hotline that can put you in touch with whatever support is available in your area. If there is none, you can seek out a church, gay organization, or the Hemophilia Foundation. *You* need to be supported yourself, and, at the same time, *you* can support another infected individual in that special way. You can even start a support group using this book as a framework, or bring this book to a preexisting group.

Share Yourself with Others

Sharing your experience, strength, and hope with someone is life enhancing. If your words fall on deaf ears, just try someone else. Don't waste your energy on someone who is unwilling to go through what you had to go through to get this far. In doing so you would be denying your support to another person who is willing to do the work.

Keep in mind that not all people are ready or willing to accept responsibility for themselves. That's not a judgment, just a fact. But you are, or you wouldn't have gotten this far in this book. There are others like you. (Having a sense of personal responsibility for one's health and a sense that one can influence one's health is another characteristic of long-term survivors.) You can search out others like you and share yourselves with each other.

Twelfth-Step Affirmations

Today I know that I can choose to be of service.

Today I choose to help another who has HIV or is at risk of developing it.

Today I want to open my heart to someone who is suffering.

Today I can choose to call another and offer my help.

Today I choose to live my life by the principles of the twelve steps.

Today I am grateful for my spiritual awakening.

Today I choose to practice the twelve-step principles in all my affairs.

Final Thoughts

We suggest you continue to use the steps and exercises on a daily basis, be true to yourself, and follow the advice of your health care professional. You can live your life, one day at a time, happy, joyous, and free. We would like to know how this program is working for you and if there is any other way we can be of help. Please let us know. We really want to hear how you are doing and help in any way we can. God bless you.

The following are the promises of the twelve-step program as described in the "Big Book" of Alcoholics Anonymous. Remember these promises and may you feel your Higher Power with you through all the days of your life.

THE PROMISES

We are going to know a new freedom and a new happiness.
We will not regret the past nor wish to shut the door on it.
We will comprehend the word serenity *and we will know peace.*
No matter how far down the scale we have gone, we will see how our experience can benefit others.
That feeling of uselessness and self-pity will slip away.
Our whole attitude and outlook upon life will change.
Fear of people and of economic insecurity will leave us.
We will intuitively know how to handle situations which used to baffle us.
We will suddenly realize that God is doing for us what we could not do for ourselves.
Are these extravagant promises?
We think not.
They are being fulfilled among us—sometimes quickly, sometimes slowly.
They will always *materialize if we work for them.*

THIRTEEN

Getting on with Living
While Dealing with the Issues of Dying

Cindy's Story

At the age of seventeen, I began having pain in the lower left side of my abdomen when I ovulated. I was a student nurse, so I soon determined that my ovary was the source of the pain.

On one particular day the pain became so bad that it radiated down my leg, making me limp as I walked. Despite my protest of virginity, the doctor responsible for the student nurses' health care insisted that I had gonorrhea and gave me an injection of penicillin.

The pain continued for three days, getting worse, when suddenly I found myself in the operating room. A cyst on one of my ovaries had caused one of my fallopian tubes to twist on itself, and, in so doing, had cut off its own blood supply. My ovary, fallopian tube, and part of my uterus had become gangrenous and had to be removed. I was in shock in the operating room and when I emerged was placed on the critical list.

I spent one day in the intensive care unit and was then sent to the regular nursing floor. I was still very weak and barely conscious. I would wake up and find that I had vomit in my mouth and hair. I was afraid that I was going to vomit while I was unconscious and choke. I called the nurse and asked her to please put a tube in my stomach to drain off the contents, so I would stop vomiting. I explained to her that I was afraid that I was going to choke.

Suddenly I found myself weightlessly hovering over my own

body. The room was filled with an unusual kind of white light, much like moonlight. All that I remember feeling was sense of awe. It felt like, All right! This is great! I remember thinking curiously, What is going on? Whatever it is, it's incredible!

I watched as the doctors and nurses worked on my body, but felt no attachment to it. It never even occurred to me to be frightened! My only feeling continued to be one of wonder and amazement.

I could see the crash cart, a cart containing the equipment that was used to resuscitate patients who had suffered a respiratory or cardiac arrest. I could also see that one doctor was doing something to my head and another one was trying to start an IV in my left ankle. I saw the nurse I had earlier asked to help me hurrying around my bed in a frenzy. Still I felt no fear, only pure astonishment and bliss. I recognized the body as mine, but was not afraid for it.

Then suddenly I felt as if some incredibly heavy force took me over. I felt so bulky, full, and heavy. Then I realized someone was doing something to my right arm. I looked up and saw the same nurse. I thought, My God, I'm in my body again! I hadn't even realized how weightless I had been until I felt the constriction and heaviness of being back in my body. I had no thoughts, just feelings—and they were pure rage! "What are you doing?" I mumbled to the nurse. I was shocked at how weak my voice sounded. She said, "I'm trying to get a blood pressure." I suddenly felt very depressed. "Just get it and leave me alone!" I heard myself say. My voice sounded very far away.

I woke up three days later and eventually found out that I had, in fact, choked on my vomit, and my breathing and heart had stopped. I told no one about my experience because I thought I had hallucinated. Since my experience much has been written about near-death experiences, and I have come to know that many other people have had experiences similar to mine. I still don't know if my experience was a hallucination. But one thing I do know is that since that time death has held no fear for me.

After graduating from nursing school I worked with the critically ill for more than fourteen years. I was at the bedsides of more than one thousand people as they too "left their bodies." My colleagues and my family always marveled at how easily I dealt with death and how supportive I was to my patients and their families. I believe my capacity to be therapeutic in these death and dying situations is a result of my own experience. Because I have already "died" myself and found my experience to be very positive, I am free to be there for my patients, unencumbered by my own fears. Once you've "died" there really are few big deals in life. Still, from time to time, despite my experience, I can get all caught up in it and forget that.

I tell you this story because it continues to comfort me, and because we know that it is difficult to think of HIV infection without also thinking about the possibility of premature death. Our research and experience leads us to believe that many of you who make good use of this type of positive program and your particular medical regime will increase your survival time enough for science to find a more specific treatment or prevention of HIV infection and AIDS. Advances are being made daily. Now, for example, with pentamadine mist, the pneumonia that frequently took the lives of many infected persons can be avoided. Nevertheless we also believe that it is important for you to address some discomfiting, perhaps disturbing, issues.

"But," you may ask, "If this is a life-affirming program, why must I entertain any thought of dying?" That's a good question. Here's how we look at it. When we drive we do not expect to have an accident, yet we wear our seat belts and ask those riding with us to wear theirs, so that in case of an accident, we are less likely to be severely injured. We do not believe that our putting on seat belts will draw an accident to us. As a matter of fact, we believe it is an act of prudence. Indeed, with all the statistics proving the efficacy of seat belts, to *not* put on a seat belt is a form of denial.

Similarly, for anyone to deny the possibility of death is not positive thinking, but denial. The person in denial creates for himself or herself an unreal world. This act of denying the fact that we will all die and leave our physical bodies someday consumes much energy, while that which is being denied creates an internal tension that is harmful physically, mentally, emotionally, and spiritually. It takes energy to deny reality. Once you confront reality and deal with it, the tension is released. That internal tension that wasted so much energy denying the possibility of death can now be freed up to work for you.

The long-term survivors we have talked to tell us that they are prepared to die but choose not to spend their lives always fearing their death. They do not feel that fear of death is a good enough reason to want to go on living. They do not believe their infection with HIV is terminal, yet it brings to their minds how precious life really is. Because of this they have made a decision to live each day as if it is a gift. They choose to live by the AA slogan "One day at a time." Yet by confronting this issue they are doing the footwork necessary to be responsible for their eventual deaths. As one person put it, "I chose to confront the issues of dying in order to live long and live well."

Several mentioned that they actually thought of how they might die and how they would like to die until they could feel comfortable with the idea. They thought of all their unfinished business—things they wanted to do and things they wanted to say—and then went and did them. They now spend their time doing things that feed their emotions and their spirits. Although not all of them are in twelve-step programs, they have, in one way or another, worked the twelve steps in various other processes and continue to live by these principles in their daily lives.

I have had a final will for many years. I know that someday I will really die and not come back into my body. We all do; it's part of the experience of all living things. I want to be sure that my last wishes are clearly stated and respected. I do not want to leave my family and friends confused and trying to guess what I would have wanted done with my body and my possessions. I have seen this happen to families far too many times. It is very hard on everyone involved. I choose to avoid that by having a will.

I also have a living will, designating what kind of care I want should something happen that keeps me from communicating my desires for treatment. Probably my working in intensive care units prompted me to draw one up. Obviously I have not needed either the final will or the living will to date, so my making them did not in any way hasten my death. I just consider what I did a reasonable and responsible thing to do.

My sponsor recently died. She had a "little" cancer but was in no way terminally ill. Before her surgery I asked her if she wanted to make out a living will. She did, and named me responsible for her medical decisions in case she became too ill to make them herself. She died shortly after a second surgery. I was able to see to it that she died in the way she had requested: no more surgeries and no life support. Because I was not related to her, without the living will I could not have made those decisions for her, and her wishes would not have been carried out.

I focus on living, but in doing so I take the steps, I do the footwork, to guarantee that things go smoothly if a catastrophic illness occurs and also for when I die. Most of the people we interviewed who have HIV infection or AIDS feel the same way. Quite a few of them have been infected for many years, and they do not consider it morbid to have wills, nor do they expect to die soon. They merely accept that HIV infection or AIDS has made them more aware of their mortality. They want to make sure things go the way they want whenever they do become terminally ill and die—as we all must one day do.

If you have not already done so, we recommend that you draw up both a written living will and a written final will. If you need help with this, please get it. Call your local AIDS hotline for the name of someone in your area who specializes in this aspect of the law. This is not focusing on death. It is living in a responsible manner, the way we know any of you reading this book want to live.

FOURTEEN

To All Significant Others

Your loved one is probably at risk of developing or is infected with the human immunodeficiency virus, HIV, or has AIDS or an HIV-related condition. We want to acknowledge you for reading this chapter. The fact that you are reading these words means that you care and are willing to explore ways you can support your loved one. You have our admiration and our prayers. Probably the question you are asking most often is, "How can I help?" Here are some suggestions.

Understanding this Program and Developing Your Support System

First of all, it will be helpful for you to read the introduction to this book, as well as Chapter 15, "To the Health Care Provider." These discuss the philosophy of this program. To be of help to your loved one while he or she is working a twelve-step program such as this one, it is best if you have an understanding of what a twelve-step program is and how it works.

Additionally, it is essential that you develop a support system for yourself. Your loved one will be unlikely to share his or her concerns with you if he or she thinks it would be too great a burden. Your loved one needs to know that you have ways to take care of yourself.

Participating in Al-Anon or a twelve-step program for people involved with someone who is at risk or is infected with HIV would be the most helpful. There you can learn how to detach with love and how to support your loved one without assuming unhealthy responsibility for him or her. Additionally, if you are in a twelve-step support group while your loved one is using a twelve-step program, you will have a common reference point for dealing with this difficult situation and for communicating with each other. The nature of your relationship will determine the manner in which you can best be of support now.

Consider reading this book in its entirety, carrying out the exercises, using the tapes, and exploring the affirmations that are appropriate to you. This basic process is a spiritual and a psychological one from which both you and your loved one can benefit.

HIV Infection and AIDS Information

Being at risk for becoming infected with HIV does not mean that one will become infected! There are many things that can be done to minimize risk and remain free of infection.

Further, being infected with HIV is not the same thing as having AIDS. True, it is believed that AIDS is caused by H IV, but most people infected with HIV do *not* have AIDS! There are many things that can be done to slow the progression of HIV infection and possibly prevent full-blown AIDS!

Even among those who do have AIDS, the disease expresses itself differently in different people. The disease presents itself in various forms, and people respond to the disease in a variety of ways. There are many things that can be done to alter the course of the disease and to stay healthy for a very long time.

Transmission Information

For your own peace of mind it's important that you understand how HIV is transmitted. Certain body fluids contain enough virus to potentially cause infection. They are: sperm, blood, vaginal secretions, breast milk, and any body fluid that has blood in it. That is why unprotected sex (see Chapter 2) and sharing IV needles are the most common ways people become infected. Essentially then, other than avoiding unsafe sex and needle sharing all you need do is: 1) wear gloves when handling anything wet with fluids from your loved one; 2) protect your mucous membranes (eyes, mouth, vagina or rectum) from these fluids, and; 3) do not share razors, toothbrushes, or sex toys.

Remember that AIDS stands for Acquired Immune Deficiency Syndrome. The human immunodeficiency virus, HIV, can cause a weakness in the immune system of an infected person. As a result, organisms that are incapable of producing disease in a healthy person can cause infection in a person with a depressed immune system. This kind of infection is called an opportunistic infection because the organism uses the *opportunity* of the suppressed immune system and an infection results. *It is the infected person who might be at risk of becoming sick from you, rather than you being likely to get an infection from him or her.* Because his or her immune system is affected, it is important that you wear a mask and avoid kissing if you are ill with something highly contagious, such as the flu or a cold.

HIV infection, however, is not contagious like a cold or the flu. You cannot get it from someone coughing on you, or from drinking out of the same glass. Nor can you get an opportunistic infection from the infected person, unless your own immune system is also severely damaged. Even mothers who have taken care of very sick infected infants have not become infected and there is probably no closer contact than that of a mother to her infant. *It is perfectly safe to hug, kiss, massage, and hold someone who is infected with HIV or has AIDS.*

An exception to this rule is the case of an HIV-infected person who has pulmonary tuberculosis, TB. TB is becoming common among HIV-infected minorities and IV drug users. TB is contagious *to* anyone. To protect yourself if your loved one has TB you need to wear a mask and glasses to protect the mucous membranes of your mouth and eyes or have the infected person wear a mask when you have close contact. It is possible to catch TB from anyone who has it and is coughing.

If you have any other questions regarding transmission of HIV or AIDS, call someone to get an informed, accurate answer. Do not ask friends or neighbors; ask someone who knows the facts.

Detachment

It is important to know how to detach yourself in relationships of any sort, but perhaps even more important in relationships where one or both people are infected with HIV. Detaching means to remain compassionate and yet not assume responsibility for someone else's feelings, behavior, or experience of reality. Because so much in a person's life is affected by this disease, it is common for the infected person to have varied responses and mood swings. As you are probably very well aware, we often take things out on the ones closest to us. For this reason it is vital that you realize that *you have control over and are responsible for only one person on this planet, and that person is you.*

Your loved one is responsible for his or her own feelings, behaviors, and experience of reality. If, in his or her anguish, he or she tries to blame you or take anger out on you, you need to realize that this is exactly what is happening. If you weren't there, someone else would likely be the target. It is important for you to accept that, and try to not take it personally. You can choose to accept responsibility for your loved one's feelings and go on a guilt trip if you wish. But you can be in only one place at a time. You can either be off on a guilt trip *or* you can be supporting your loved one. It is up to you!

If you do not know how to detach yourself, this will be very difficult. No matter how many times you may have heard "You make me _____," it is not true! Short of holding a gun to your head, as an adult no one can make you feel, do, or believe anything unless you allow it. It is a choice. Sometimes the choice is an unconscious one, so it certainly doesn't *feel* like a choice, but it is a choice nonetheless. It is a choice to feel guilty, to feel mad, to feel sad, and so on.

Likewise, *you cannot control or cure your loved one.* If he or she feels, says, or does something that you do not agree with, it is not your responsibility to try to change him or her. You need to "take a first step" on your loved one. That means accepting that you are powerless over him or her. What he or she feels, thinks, says, or does is up to him or her. You did not *cause* his or her disease, thoughts, feelings, or actions. (Even if your loved one was infected through contact with you, it was probably the result of an act your partner consented to of his or her own free will. Your feeling guilty and upset now will not help your loved one or yourself.)

This situation is incredibly difficult. Because the virus can affect a person's mind it may make the situation even more difficult. It's not right to hold anyone accountable when his or her mind is affected. He or she may not mean what he or she says or does at all. *It may be the HIV disease talking.* And you can be angry at the disease rather than the person. But you are still not responsible for what he or she feels, thinks, or does. If you were to accept that responsibility you would lessen your own chance of being of any help to yourself or your loved ones. Neither can you *control* or *cure* his or her disease, feelings, thoughts, or actions. These are the three Cs of Al-Anon. You didn't *cause* it, and you can't *control* or *cure* it.

At the same time you need to be true to yourself. There are many cofactors that seem to affect the outcome of this infection. If you think that something that your loved one is doing is not in his or her best interests, such as drinking alcohol or using drugs, it is your right and responsibility to say so—*once.* But *understand that your loved one's behavior is his or her responsibility, not yours!* All you can do is state your concern; your responsibility ends there. Nagging won't help, as millions of partners and relatives of alcoholics and addicts can tell you.

It is important, however, to remain true to yourself. If you can't stand to watch what your loved one is doing to himself or herself, you don't have to. You might need to set limits and boundaries. If you can't find a place of detachment that gives you the comfort you need, you can certainly state your case and leave. Some partners of alcoholics or addicts make the decision that certain behaviors are taboo. They will not, for example, ride in the car, share a bed, or stay in public with a partner when he or she is under the influence. Others find the entire situation unbearable and separate from or divorce their partners. Many factors are at play here, including how abusive the person may become. But the bottom line is you have the right and the responsibility to take care of yourself, whatever that takes.

It Is Your Loved One's Life!

Keep in mind that there are many ways people choose to respond to this disease. Some long-term AIDS or HIV survivors eat a very strict diet, others eat everything they want. Some take medication prescribed by their doctor, others take no traditional drugs. Some strictly monitor their immune function, others don't know and don't care what their immune status is.

Your loved one may choose to respond to this disease in a manner with which you do not agree. All of us who are parents certainly know the feeling of frustration when our children take paths different from the ones we would have picked for them. Sometimes we have to stand by and watch unbelievable tragedies. Detachment is the only hopeful and sane way for you to survive and be of true value to anyone.

There are now available a wide variety of traditional medical management and various holistic therapies, such as massage and acupuncture, as well as emotional counseling and support groups. But it is important for the infected person to make his or her own decisions about how to respond to this disease. *He or she may not want to do it your way.* Please honor that! It is important that he or she make his or her own decisions, even if you do not agree. Try to support your loved one regardless of what approach he or she chooses. Ultimately, it is his or her body and life!

Emotional Responses

There are certain predictable emotional responses to this infection. Most people at risk of developing HIV, those already infected with HIV, and those who have AIDS, as well as their family, other loved ones, and friends, go through these stages. *Keep in mind that you too will be going through these stages.* They are not fixed in order or in time, so people may go in and out of the various stages at various times. You may even revert back to certain stages as time goes on and circumstances change.

These stages include anxiety, denial, focusing on imagined symptoms (somatization), anger, depression, and acceptance. This twelve-step program addresses all of these stages.

Anxiety

The best approach for handling your anxiety is to gather information, do relaxation exercises, and join a support group, such as a twelve-step group—perhaps Al-Anon—or whatever other spiritual group you find helpful, and live your life by its principles.

Some of the ways you can support your loved one's response to anxiety is to be there to listen (you don't have to have answers), direct him or her to information and support groups, support functional and active problem solving, participate in relaxation exercises and healthy diversionary activities, emphasize staying in the present moment, and provide nonsexual touch, such as back rubs and hugs.

What about Denial?

Don't try arguing with denial. If your loved one or you need to deny, respect that need. The mind uses denial until it can handle reality. Denial is usually temporary, and the first step in this program works toward overcoming damaging denial. It would be appropriate, however, to intervene and try to break through dangerous denial that poses a threat to your loved one, yourself, or others. Keep in mind, however, that the decision regarding his or her behavior is ultimately up to him or her. You cannot control his or her behavior, no matter how good your intention.

Accepting the infection or the diagnosis, but refusing to accept that he or she will die from it, is a very healthy kind of denial, and *a real possibility.* There are people who have lived long and lived well with this disease! This kind of denial—denial of the worst-case scenario—is commonly found in long-term survivors of many life-threatening diseases. It is life enhancing and can provide the impetus for searching out and experiencing many of the various healing strategies that can heal not only the body, but also the mind, emotions, and spirit.

Focusing on Every Little Symptom

The best way to deal with somatization (too much attention to meaningless physical symptoms, on the part of either you or your loved one) is to seek out medical interpretation of the symptom. Again, you want to support *focusing on action*. Worrying about whether a dark spot is a bruise or a Kaposi's lesion can drive both of you crazy. We suggest you support your loved one in getting a professional medical opinion, or get one yourself.

While waiting for that opinion, stay in the present moment. What can be done about it right now, right this very second? If nothing, then do something to get your mind off of it. You can call someone who has been through something similar; go to a movie or for a walk, sing a song, scrub the tile in the bathroom, write about it, take a shower, listen to a meditation tape, do anything constructive—but don't just sit there! Do something! Move your muscles and change your thoughts.

Anger and Depression

Most anger is born of fear, and until you or your loved one becomes deeply entrenched in the philosophy of a twelve-step or some other spiritual program, both of you may take your anger out on each other. This is why learning to detach yourself is so very important.

Remember that you too will be going through these stages. You are also powerless over the infection and powerless over your loved one. But you are not powerless over how you will respond to either. You have a choice. You can buy into the anger and get yourself all upset and maybe even get sick yourself. Then you'd be of less value to your loved one and yourself. Or you can work through your anger, and detach from your loved one's anger. You really didn't *cause* your loved one's anger, and you can't *control* it or *cure* it. Remembering these Three Cs will help you keep things in perspective. But it will be exceedingly difficult, if not impossible, to do it alone. Try getting into a program yourself, for your own good and the good of your loved one.

Acceptance

Acceptance is very tricky. Acceptance of the specfic stage you or your loved one is in is important. Only with acceptance can appropriate action be taken. Each person comes to acceptance in his or her own time. You may come to acceptance before or after your loved one does. If you two are in different stages of acceptance, try to respect where you both are. Avoid judging one as right and one as wrong. There is really no right or wrong; there is only different.

Acceptance is not the same thing as giving up. Giving up is despair, and despair is very detrimental to physical, mental, emotional, and spiritual well-being. Acceptance involves being aware of whatever stage of the diagnosis a person is in. Out of that awareness, a person can act in whatever way is appropriate. He or she could have blood tests, take medication, follow specific diets, take naps, have acupuncture, go to therapy, meditate, visualize, and so on. *But in doing so, that person can still continue to go forward with life.*

If Your Loved One Became Infected from Nonsexual or Nondrug-Related Behaviors

Even though your loved one's way of life might be quite different from that of the larger population of people infected with HIV, this program can work just as well. In fact, we believe everyone on the planet could be helped if they lived their lives by the principles of the twelve steps. So the twelve steps can be effective for him or her, and you too, if you work them. Likewise, although a few of the statements in this chapter may not relate to you or your loved ones, most of them do. You will feel the same feelings, maybe even more so. You may be even more inclined to feel justified in blaming and projecting out your anger on a really unfair situation.

Regardless of how your loved one became infected, the dynamics of living with that infection are the same. And the dynamics of how you can be of most support are the same. So please read on and use what applies, while leaving out that which does not. And please get some support for yourself! This is a long, tough journey you are both on, and you will find it easier if you don't try to do it alone. This is a time for heroes, not martyrs.

If Your Loved One Is Your Daughter or Son

This can be one of the most excruciatingly painful situations of your life. Watching your child, no matter what his or her age, go through a difficult time is often as hard on the parent as it is on the child. But remember that if you get stuck in guilt over this, you will be of little help to anyone. Do whatever you need to do to get out of self-absorbed guilt if you really want to help your son or daughter.

If your child is at risk of infection or infected with HIV owing to some behavior that you do not approve of, this is going to be very difficult, *but* this is certainly not the time to give sermons or pass judgment. *Your child needs your unconditional love and support now more than perhaps ever before!* If you find that you are unable to be nonjudgmental, but want to be of help, then please get counseling to work thorugh your issues. This is an unbelievably difficult situation for everyone involved. Please be gentle with yourself, your spouse, and your child.

If your child has not lived at home for some time and you don't know his or her friends very well, please try to be courteous. It's very sad to watch friends who have been a person's major emotional support for perhaps years suddenly pushed away and not even allowed to visit their loved one because of angry parents. For this very reason many people do not tell their parents about their infection until it is far advanced. Both the parents and the child suffer in this case. Your coming to terms with your judgments can help. You can still love your child without loving his or her way of life, no matter what that may be. Difficult, yes—but impossible, no.

This is no time to ask your child to choose between parents and partner or friends. Your child needs all the support he or she can get from everyone who loves him or her. It's very easy at times to be overcome by the magnitude of this illness and, out of anger and shame, scapegoat somebody, anybody, to ease the pain. That's why it's so valuable for you too to have a support group where you can air these kinds of feelings and find assistance in dealing with these difficult issues. This can be a time of healing for the whole family if you let it. It is your choice.

If Your Loved One Is Your Brother, Sister, Mother, or Father

Everything we mentioned to parents also applies to you. If it is your brother or sister who is at risk or is infected with HIV, you know how much he or she needs your support. If you were abused as a child, read about codependency and abuse. Your loved one is so lucky to have you!

If the person at risk or infected is one of your parents, and if he or she became infected through sexual or drug activity, this can be a most painful challenge for you. You may find yourself so filled with resentment, anger, and grief that you don't know what to do first. The chapter on codependency and abuse will be helpful. There are also support groups, such as Adult Children of Alcoholics, that can help you sort through your relationship with your parent. Your parent does not have to be an alcoholic for you to be helped in this group. A person from any type of dysfunctional family can find support there.

If you can come to a place of forgiveness and finally compassion for your parent, you will both experience a wonderful healing. *It is never too late.* It will require a great deal of work on both of your parts, but the fact that you are even reading this page says that you are certainly willing and trying to do just that. Just your being there for your parent will mean so much. With help you can choose to be there for your parent, even if you do not feel he or she has been there for you.

If Your Loved One Is Your Partner or Spouse

In addition to everything that we have already mentioned, it is important for you to protect yourself by having only safe sex. This may or may not be a hard thing to do, depending on the nature of your relationship. If you find that it is difficult, then you need to reread step two. You need to find a way to be assertive enough so that you can insist on safe sex. Do not think that just because you have not developed an HIV-positive test so far that you are not going to. Please protect yourself. Only you can.

It will also be extremely important for you to join a support group, such as Al-Anon. Because your relationship is one where you are intimately involved on a daily basis with your loved one, you will be the one most affected by his or her HIV status and emotional and physical health. It will also be you whom your loved one will turn to most for emotional and other types of support. You can give only what you've got. You must continuously replenish your supply of strength by seeking outside support and counsel.

It is vital that you attempt to stay physically, mentally, emotionally, and spiritually fit. You can do that only by taking very good care of yourself. This is not the time to play self-sacrificing martyr. To do so would hurt not only you, but also your loved one. When he or she needs you the most you might find that your cup is empty unless you take good care of yourself and let others help so you can rest and refill your cup.

It is also more important for you to learn the art of detachment. You are affected on a daily basis by the demands of this condition and may be used as a whipping post by your loved one. Make sure that you take time out for yourself and set limits on what you will do and accept. You may be used to always putting others first, but that can be very detrimental. Read the section on codependency and Chapter 2. You, as well as your loved one, may need to learn more about becoming assertive. It is possible to support your loved one and still take good care of yourself. But you have to have permission from yourself to do that. A support group will help you give yourself that permission.

Our compassion and prayers go out to you. We hope this chapter has been helpful in some way.

FIFTEEN

To the Health Care Provider

Why a Chapter to the Health Care Provider?

We address this chapter to you, the health care provider, so that you can become knowledgeable and comfortable with this program and thereby more easily support your patient or client in his or her use of a twelve-step approach to his or her infection with HIV. We encourage you to read the entire book, especially Chapter 1, with its many references, but realize that you may not have time. Therefore, if you contact us we will send you chapter summaries, so that you can discuss your patients' work with them in an informed fashion.

Unique Challenges Posed by HIV Infection

The disease believed to be caused by the human immuno-deficiency virus, HIV, offers some unique challenges. The normal method of prevention of most infectious diseases has historically been by vaccination. Most other infectious diseases for which preventive vaccines do not exist are usually self-limiting or treatable by rest, antibiotics, and symptomatic medication. As you well know, that is not the case with HIV infection.

Despite several years of research, no vaccine for the prevention of HIV infection has thus far been found, and most researchers do not expect to find a single medical cure for those already infected or those who have already progressed to AIDS. Yet as we know, AIDS is a severely disabling and potentially fatal disease.

Unique to HIV infection is the long latency period in most individuals from infection to the development of clinical illness. Even more troublesome is the fact that infected individuals who have no clinical symptoms remain contagious to others.

Another burden on the health care system is the fact that most of the population at risk, especially in developed countries, comes from minority groups that have long been alienated from mainstream society. Furthermore, behavior change, not an easy task, is one of the few supportive activities that a person at risk of developing HIV or already infected with HIV can do to prevent infection and illness (or further infection and illness) to himself or herself, as well as transmission to others.

Thus when we consider the enormous distress related to infection, the ambiguity of treatment and outcome, the oppressive conditions of minority groups, the even further prejudice and social ostracism that befall infected individuals, and the crucial need to prevent further spread of infection, we can see clearly why the role of the traditional health care provider is stretched beyond previous limits.

Challenges to the Mental Health Care Provider

The role of the mental health care provider is of paramount importance throughout the entire spectrum of this disease. Mental and emotional distress spans from the worried well individuals who are anxious about, but not infected with HIV, to the individuals in terminal stages of full-blown AIDS, as well as all of their loved ones.

HIV infection, however, presents a very special challenge to the mental health care provider. You have probably never before been asked to work with as many clients who have problems related to a potentially life-threatening infectious disease. You may, in addition, feel ill equipped to work with the minority groups that often make up this special patient population.

It is our intention to provide for the person at risk of developing HIV or infected with HIV, as well as for the health care provider and the mental health care provider working with such individuals, a simple model to assist them in dealing with these challenges.

It is also our hope that clinicians working with substance abuse patients in or out of treatment centers will see how this model for dealing with HIV infection can easily be used for their patients. In this way those who work with substance abusers can learn to deal with HIV infection, and those who work with HIV-infected people can learn to deal with substance abuse.

HIV and substance abuse must be looked at together. And yet we find many clinicians, for whatever reasons, reluctant to deal with both issues. We hope this book can be of assistance.

A twelve-step model for substance abuse can easily be shifted to encompass the risk of, or infection with HIV. We believe treatment centers are one of the best possible places for high-risk clients to be educated, tested, and supported. Leaving a treatment center still wondering whether one is infected is certainly not conducive to long-term sobriety. Treatment centers who test patients find that it does not lead to increased relapse when handled by a well-trained counselor who is not in personal fear. As a matter of fact, for most high-risk clients, it can prevent relapse.[1,2] We also believe clinicians treating infected individuals are in a unique position to help their patients face and begin to deal with substance abuse (see Chapter 1's references).

Rationale and General Description:
A Twelve-Step Program

This program is based on the twelve-step program originally developed by the cofounders of Alcoholics Anonymous. We have expanded it to gently address the behavioral, psychological, and human spirit needs of the population at risk or infected with HIV. For more than fifty years these twelve steps have proven effective for various groups of people who too have, in one way or another, felt alienated and estranged from society at large. As you are probably well aware, they have been modified and used by many groups, including Al-Anon, Adult Children of Alcoholics, Overeaters Anonymous, Codependents Anonymous, Narcotics Anonymous, Sex and Love Addicts Anonymous, Prostitutes Anonymous, Cocaine Anonymous, and more.

Our rationale for selecting this approach is that experience and research indicate that the same dynamics present in substance abusers are also present in persons infected with HIV. Infected individuals seem to undergo the same kind of denial and self-hatred; feelings of hopelessness, helplessness, and alienation; and sense of being overwhelmed by something beyond their control.

Society also tends to be morally judgmental of, lack understanding of, and ostracize both those who are substance abusers and those who are infected with HIV. Needless to say, the biggest risk groups for HIV infection, gay and bisexual men and IV drug addicts, historically have had to deal with these issues long before the advent of HIV.

Additionally, perhaps partly owing to these psychic stressors as well as to genetic factors and the frequent use of bars for socialization, the rate of alcohol and drug abuse in the homosexual population has consistently been reported to be three times that of the rest of society (see Chapter 1's references). Unfortunately, this problem is frequently unaddressed in the HIV-infected patient, which only leads to further high-risk behavior, depression, and suicide.[3] The likelihood of alcohol abuse in a parent of an HIV-infected person is also very high.

Therefore, if you add the subpopulation of gay and bisexuals who are infected and who are also substance abusers to the IV drug addict population, and if you also add in the heterosexual and pediatric populations who are infected via the IV drug addict route, it becomes clear that the major risk factor for HIV infection is substance abuse!

This is an important part of our rationale for the use of the twelve-step model, which has, over time, proven to be uniquely suited to and effective with this type of population.

Dr. Stuart Nichols describes the specific effectiveness of a support group based on the model of Alcoholics Anonymous for people infected with HIV.

> In the group, patients learn to take responsibility for their own reactions. . . . They help each other identify unreasonableness . . . thoughts which color their response. . . . They learn that, while they must accept the conditions that AIDS imposes, they still have the ability to control their attitudes, make their own decisions, and

manage their lives. . . . Concomitantly, patients scruti-
nize the quality of their lives, conducting a fearless
examination for the sources of pain and pleasure. They
consider almost everything that touches their existence.
. . . They learn to dismiss the quick fix. . . . Individuals
are encouraged to be scrupulously honest. *As a result,
values and behavior can change rapidly.* . . . Patients
encourage one another to live each day to the fullest
. . . report they feel more vibrant, spiritual, spontaneous,
and content . . . had not imagined such a state of alive-
ness was possible before AIDS. They spend considerable
time in helping others. . . . This is a remarkable transfor-
mation. . . . Psychiatrists should benefit from familiarity
with this remarkable phenomenon.[4]

Others report the specific effectiveness of the twelve-step approach in reducing unsafe sexual practices and as a framework for
people with AIDS (PWAs) to use in dealing with HIV infection in
the context of an alcohol or drug recovery program.[5, 6]

It is our feeling that the support and self-acceptance inherent
in working a twelve-step program provide a foundation on which
persons at risk or infected with HIV can build a strong and healthy
mental, emotional, and spiritual base for themselves, as well as
developing strategies for coping actively with the multidimensional
challenge of HIV.[7-11]

Dr. George Solomon of the University of California, Los
Angeles, and Lydia Temoshok, Ph.D., of the University of California, San Francisco, have been studying long-term survivors,
people who have had AIDS for several years. They report the
one most consistent finding that correlates with positive immune
measurements is "the ability to say no to an unwanted favor,
reflecting assertiveness, lack of masochism and self-sacrifice, and
the ability to take care of oneself." They also noted that the
following characteristics were frequently found in long-term survivors they studied. Our experience and research verifies these
findings.

A long-term survivor:

1. Perceives the treating physician as a collaborator, and does not interact with him or her in either a passive or a defiant mode.

2. Has a sense of personal responsibility for his or her own health and a sense that he or she can influence it.

3. Has a commitment to his or her life in terms of unfinished business, unmet goals, or unfulfilled wishes.

4. Has a sense of purpose in life.

5. Finds new meaning as a result of the illness itself.

6. Has previously mastered a life-threatening illness or other life crisis.

7. Engages in a physical fitness or exercise program.

8. Derives useful information from, and has supportive contact with, a person with AIDS soon after his or her own diagnosis.

9. Is altruistically involved with other AIDS patients.

10. Has accepted the reality of the diagnosis of AIDS, yet refuses to perceive the condition as a death sentence.

11. Has an ability to communicate his or her concerns, including those regarding the illness.

12. Is assertive and has the ability to say no.

13. Has the ability to withdraw from involvements and to nurture himself or herself.

14. Is sensitive to his or her body and its needs.

We realize that this information is observational only, and not from a controlled study of AIDS patients chosen at random, but the findings are similar to other findings related to attitudes and longevity in studies on patients with other life-threatening disease.[12-16] We also believe these characteristics would benefit patients in attaining a better quality of life during any life-threatening illness, regardless of its outcome. The twelve-step process encourages the development of these characteristics and would therefore be of special value to individuals at risk or infected with HIV.

Stress Reduction, Relaxation, and Imagery Training

Often the same set of dynamics that has contributed to people being at risk or infected with HIV keeps these individuals from caring for themselves properly. Lack of coping skills and problem-solving strategies also contribute to the spread of infection and interfere with activities that support a higher quality of life and adequate self-care, which could maximize their immunological competence. Besides the twelve-step format, the other powerful aspect of this program is its use of relaxation and imagery. It is through the use of relaxation and imagery that these mal-adaptive dynamics can be most easily interrupted and replaced with healthy responses.

It has been demonstrated that certain coping styles, that is, denial, the use of drugs and alcohol, psychological distress (especially depression), absence of self-efficacy, and absence of social and emotional support, determine the continuation of high-risk activities and impede self-care.[17-26] One study of the effect of childhood sexual abuse found that those who had been sexually abused were twice as likely to work as prostitutes, with increased IV drug use; and that 33 percent of survivors of rape versus 21 percent of those never raped had evidence of HIV infection.[27]

Relaxation and imagery have proven to be beneficial for reducing stress, depression, and high-risk sexual behavior, as well as increasing the health locus of control and feelings of efficacy.[4, 28-32] Studies also suggest that relaxation and imagery may actually enhance immune function in other populations, as well as in those dealing with HIV infection.[32-40]

Relaxation and imagery, which have been very well received by this patient population, assist the patient in moving through the twelve steps with greater ease. Through the use of mental rehearsal of various behavior changes, cognitive restructuring skills, thought stopping, and other coping strategies, the patient learns active coping skills and gains a greater sense of control. Active coping and an increased sense of efficacy have been demonstrated to enhance mental and physical health, and may, in turn, influence the progression of HIV disease.[41-57]

Other active coping strategies that have been found to increase immune functioning in individuals at risk of developing HIV or infected with HIV include exercise, which is also stressed in the program.[45, 58-61]

How to Use this Program

The best use of this book is in a group setting. This program can either be brought to an existing group or a group can be built around it. We feel group interventions can be particularly helpful because they create social support among the members, reduce social isolation, and enable the client to identify with others who are dealing with the same issues, as well as provide a place for learning constructive coping strategies.[29, 49, 54-57, 62, 63] Because of the problems inherent to HIV infection and the nature of the high-risk groups, previously mentioned, we especially feel the social support found in group process is of immense value to this population.

Studies have shown that HIV-infected individuals who participate in peer groups have fewer hospital visits, engage in fewer high-risk behaviors, have less depression, and have a more integrated positive identity.[64-70] One study correlated helpfulness of peers with less anxiety and depression,[71] while other studies especially pointed to the advantages of peer groups for adolescents in increasing self-esteem and decreasing high-risk behavior.[72-75] Additionally, studies have consistently shown social support to be protective and predictive of both morbidity and mortality in a wide range of populations, even after adjustment for biomedical risk factors.[76-80]

If an individual already belongs to another twelve-step support group, this program can easily extend the twelve-step process to address the HIV-related issues not covered in the other twelve-step programs. (There are twelve-step programs that do not deal with alcohol, drugs, or sex, so that not only is the HIV infection not directly addressed, but neither are the risks posed by drug use, alcohol abuse, or unsafe sex.) Because this program covers in more specific terms issues related to HIV infection that are not part of other twelve-step programs, already belonging to another program does not eliminate the need for carrying out the processes suggested in this book.

Some individuals may choose to use this program alone or with the support of a counselor. We suggest that individuals receive counseling in addition to using this book. If this program is used without the support of a group it is even more important that the individual receive counseling. If this is impossible or impractical, the book can be used with a buddy or alone. All in all, we feel that the use of this book in any setting will be of significant value.

We also encourage you to take advantage of some type of support for yourself. You are probably already acutely aware of the professional burnout rate in those working with substance abusers or HIV-infected people.[81-84]

We are very interested in hearing how this book has worked for any of your clients or patients. Please write or call us. Our addresses and phone numbers are included in the Resources appendix. Thank you for your interest, your time, and your love.

REFERENCES

CHAPTER ONE REFERENCES

1. Lifson, A., Hessol, N., Rutherford, G., et al, *Natural History of HIV Infection in a Cohort of Homosexual and Bisexual Men: Clinical and Immunologic Outcome, 1977–1990.* Dept. Public Health, S.F.; Div. HIV/AIDS, CDC, Atlanta, GA, VIth International Conference on AIDS, San Francisco, CA (1990).

2. Lifson, A., Hessol, N., Rutherford, G., Buchbinder, S., et al, *The Natural History of HIV Infection in a Cohort of Homosexual and Bisexual Men: Clinical Manifestations, 1978–1989.* Vth International Conference on AIDS, Montreal, Canada (1989).

3. Gomperts, E., Holman, R., Jason, J., et al, *Effect of Age on AIDS Attack Rate in Hemophiliacs in California.* Vth International Conference on AIDS, Montreal, Canada (1989).

4. Augustyniak, L., Kramer, A., Fricke, W., et al, *U.S. HIV Seroconversion Surveillance Project: Regional Sero-positivity Rates for HIV Infection in Patients with Hemophilia.* National Hemophilia Foundation, N.Y., N.Y.; CDC, Atlanta, GA, VIth International Conference on AIDS, San Francisco, CA (1990).

5. Mundy, T., Lieb, L., Ward, J., Allen, F., et al, *Seven Year Follow-Up of HIV Infection in Neonatal Transfusion Recipients.* Vth International Conference on AIDS, Montreal, Canada (1989).

6. Hardy, A. (The Long-Term Survivor Study Group), *Characterization of Long-Term Survivors of AIDS: A Preliminary Report.* IVth International Conference on AIDS, Stockholm, Sweden (1988).

7. Operskalski, E. (Transfusion Safety Study Group), *Transient Anti-HIV Seropositivity.* IVth International Conference on AIDS, Stockholm, Sweden (1988).

8. Farzadegan, H., Wolinsky, S., Sninsky, J., et al, *Loss of Serologic and Virologic Markers of HIV-1 in Asymptomatic HIV-1 Infected Homosexual Men.* Vth International Conference on AIDS, Montreal, Canada (1989).

9. Thompson, J., Kapila, R., Tecson, F., *Human Immunodeficiency Infection in the Elderly: A Retrospective Analysis of 20 Patients.* Vth International Conference on AIDS, Montreal, Canada (1989).

10. Jones, D., Byers, R., Bush, T., Rogers, M., *The Epidemiology of Transfusion-Associated (TA) AIDS in Children in the United States, 1981 to 1988.* Vth International Conference on AIDS, Montreal, Canada (1989).

11. Oxtoby, M., Rogers, M., Bush, T., Berkelman, R., *National Surveillance of Perinatally-Acquired AIDS, USA.* Vth International Conference on AIDS, Montreal, Canada (1989).

12. Chamberland, M., Conley, L., Buehler, J., *Surveillance of Heterosexually Acquired AIDS, USA.* Vth International Conference on AIDS, Montreal, Canada (1989).

13. Gorter, R., Kocurek, K., Brodie, B., Bacchetti, P., et al, *Progression of HIV Disease in Intravenous Drug Users.* Vth International Conference on AIDS, Montreal, Canada (1989).

14. Anzala, Aggrey, Wambugu, P., Bosire, M., et al, *The Rate of Development of HIV-1 Related Illness in Women with a Known Duration of Infection.* VIth International Conference on AIDS, San Francisco, CA (1990).

15. Kilbourne, B., Chu, S., Oxtoby, M., Rogers, M., *Mortality Due to HIV Infection in Adolescents and Young Adults.* CDC, Atlanta, GA, VIth International Conference on AIDS, San Francisco, CA (1990).

16. Hersh, B., Byers, R., Karon, J., Buehler, J., *AIDS Mortality Trends Among Homosexual/Bisexual Men.* CDC, Atlanta, GA, VIth International Conference on AIDS, San Francisco, CA (1990).

17. Weiss, S., Denny, T., French, J., et al, *Increased Risk of AIDS in Older Intravenous Drug Abusers and Rates of HIV Seroconversion: 5-year Follow-up Findings from the New Jersey Intravenous Drug Abuser Cohort Study.* VIth International Conference on AIDS, San Francisco, CA (1990).

18. Young, M., Pierce, P., *Natural History of HIV Disease in an Urban Cohort of Women.* VIth International Conference on AIDS, San Francisco, CA (1990).

19. Berkelman, R., Fleming, P., Green, T., et al, *The Epidemic of AIDS in Intravenous Drug Users and Their Heterosexual Partners in the Southeastern United States.* VIth International Conference on AIDS, San Francisco, CA (1990).

20. Masiero, J., Chen, R., Armour, G., et al, *Second Generation of Heterosexual Transmission of HIV.* VIth International Conference on AIDS, San Francisco, CA (1990).

21. Wendell, D., Onorato, I., Allen, D., et al, *HIV Seroprevalence Among Adolescents and Young Adults in Selected Clinical Settings, United States, 1988–90.* CDC, Atlanta, GA, VIth International Conference on AIDS, San Francisco, CA (1990).

22. Kellogg, T., Marelich, W., Wilson, M., et al, *HIV Prevalence Among Homosexual and Bisexual Men in the San Francisco Bay Area: Evidence of Infection Among Young Gay Men.* VIth International Conference on AIDS, San Francisco, CA (1990).

23. Onorato, I., Peterson, L., Pappaioanou, M., Dondero, T., *Prevalence of HIV Infection in Heterosexual Persons in the United States, 1988–1989.* Vth International Conference on AIDS, Montreal, Canada (1989).

24. Kelley, P., Pomerantz, R., Wann, F., et al, *Relative Risk Estimates for HIV Seropositivity in Black Men: The Worsening Trend Among U.S. Soldiers.* VIth International Conference on AIDS, San Francisco, CA (1990).

25. Kingsley, L., Bacellar, H., Zhou, S., et al, *Temporal Trends in HIV Seroconversion. A Report from the Multicenter AIDS Cohort Study (MACS).* VIth International Conference on AIDS, San Francisco, CA (1990).

26. Allen, D., Onorato, I., Sweeney, P., et al, *Seroprevalence of HIV Infection in Intravenous Drug Users in the United States.* CDC, Atlanta, GA, VIth International Conference on AIDS, San Francisco, CA (1990).

27. Metler, R., Stehr-Green, J., *AIDS Surveillance Among American Indians and Alaskan Natives.* CDC, Atlanta, GA, VIth International Conference on AIDS, San Francisco, CA (1990).

28. Weiss, S., French, J., Holland, B., Parker, M., et al, *HTLV I/II Co-Infection is Significantly Associated with Risk for Progression to AIDS Among HIV+ Intravenous Drug Abusers.* Vth International Conference on AIDS, Montreal, Canada (1989).

29. Weber, R., Ledergerber, B., Opravil, M., Luthy, R., *Cessation of Intravenous Drug Use Reduces Progression of HIV Infection in HIV+ Drug Users.* VIth International Conference on AIDS, San Francisco, CA (1990).

30. Gorter, R., Vranizan, K., Moss, R., Brodie, B., Wolfe, H., *Progression of HIV Disease in Intravenous Drug Users.* VIth International Conference on AIDS, San Francisco, CA (1990).

31. Cooley, P., Van der Horst, C., Waskin, H., *A Model of Needle-Sharing and Sexual Transmission Effects on the Spread of HIV Infection.* IVth International Conference on AIDS, Stockholm, Sweden (1988).

32. Lake-Bakaar, G., Rao, R.S., *Alcohol and HIV Disease Progression in Intravenous Drug Addicts.* Vth International Conference on AIDS, Montreal, Canada (1989).

33. Becherer, P., White, G., McMillan, C., Lemon, S., *Hepatitis B and HIV Coinfection in Hemophiliacs.* Vth International Conference on AIDS, Montreal, Canada (1989).

34. Kaslow, R., VanRaden, M., DeLoria, M., et al, *Do Clinical Herpes Simplex Virus (HV) and Varicella-Zoster (VZV) Infections Accelerate HIV-1 Induced Immunodeficiency?* Vth International Conference on AIDS, Montreal, Canada (1989).

35. Hessol, N., Barnhart, L., O'Malley, P., et al, *The Natural History of HIV Infection in a Cohort of Homosexual and Bisexual Men: Cofactors for Disease Progression, 1978–1989.* Vth International Conference on AIDS, Montreal, Canada (1989).

36. Campbell, R., Halpin, T., Lanese, R., Para, M., *Hepatitis B and Other Predictors of HIV Infection Among Females in the Midwest United States.* VIth International Conference on AIDS, San Francisco, CA (1990).

37. Farr, W., Siddiqui, A., Judson, F., Penley, K., *Hepatitis B Virus DNA in Mononuclear Cells: A Potential Co-Factor of HIV Infection.* VIth International Conference on AIDS, San Francisco, CA (1990).

38. Borkowski, J., Albin, R., Schwartz, J., Mallon, R., *The Epstein Barr Virus (EBS) BZLF1 Gene Product Activates the HIV-1 5′ LTR.* VIth International Conference on AIDS, San Francisco, CA (1990).

39. Shibata, D., Nathwani, B., Brynes, R., Lenine, A., *Detection of Epstein-Barr Viral Sequences in Benign Lymph Node Biopsies from HIV Infected Patients and*

the Association with Lymphoma. VIth International Conference on AIDS, San Francisco, CA (1990).

40. Lee, C., Phillips, A., Elford, J., et al, *Ten Year Follow-up of a Cohort of 111 Anti-HIV Seropositive Hemophiliacs.* VIth International Conference on AIDS, San Francisco, CA (1990).

41. Thomas, G., Geraci, A., Lavigne, J., Levy, M., *Recurrent Anogenital Warts and HIV Status.* VIth International Conference on AIDS, San Francisco, CA (1990).

42. Payne, S., Lemp, G.F., Rutherford G.W., Neal D.P., Temelso, T., *Effect of Multiple Disease Manifestations on Length of Survival for AIDS Patients in San Francisco.* Vth International Conference on AIDS, Montreal, Canada (1989).

43. *HIV/AIDS Surveillance Report.* Centers for Disease Control, Atlanta, GA, July, 1990.

44. Zierler, S., Feingold, L., Laufer, D., et al, *Prevalence of HIV Infection and Distribution of Risk Factors Among Heterosexuals in Southeast New England.* VIth International Conference on AIDS, San Francisco, CA (1990).

45. Gwinn, M., George, J.R., Hannon, W., et al, *Estimates of HIV Seroprevalence in Childbearing Women and Incidence of HIV Infection in Infants, United States.* VIth International Conference on AIDS, San Francisco, CA (1990).

46. Moran, J., Peterman, T., Gershman, K., et al, *Gonorrhea and Syphilis Trends During the AIDS Epidemic: USA.* VIth International Conference on AIDS, San Francisco, CA (1990).

47. Wiebel, W., Lampinen, T., Chene, D., Stevko, B., *HIV-1 Seroconversion in a Cohort of Street Intravenous Drug Users in Chicago.* VIth International Conference on AIDS, San Francisco, CA (1990).

48. Beeker, C., Rose, D., Thomas, Ames L., *Marginal Men. Mainstream Risk.* VIth International Conference on AIDS, San Francisco, CA (1990).

49. Abramowitz, A., Guydish, J., Woods, W., Clark, W., *Trends in Crack Use in an AIDS Epicenter: San Francisco, 1986–1989.* VIth International Conference on AIDS, San Francisco, CA (1990).

50. Bastien, A., DeHovitz, J., Covino, J.M., et al, *Risk Factors for HIV Infection in an Urban Hospital Based STD Clinic.* VIth International Conference on AIDS, San Francisco, CA (1990).

51. Golden, D., Fullilove, M., Fullilove, R., et al, *The Effects of Gender and Crack Use on High Risk Behaviors.* VIth International Conference on AIDS, San Francisco, CA (1990).

52. Saint, Cyr-Delpe, *Update to the Community Response on Women and AIDS.* Vth International Conference on AIDS, Montreal, Canada (1989).

53. Koch, T., Jeremy, R., Lewis, E., et al, *Developmental Abnormalities in Uninfected Infants Born to HIV Infected Mothers.* VIth International Conference on AIDS, San Francisco, CA (1990).

54. Lasley-Bibbs, V., Renzullo, P., Goldenbaum, M., et al, *Patterns of Pregnancy and Reproductive Morbidity among HIV-Infected Women in the United States Army: A Retrospective Cohort Study.* VIth International Conference on AIDS, San Francisco, CA (1990).

55. Biggar, R.J., Pahwa, S., Landesman, S., et al, *Helper and Suppressor Lymphocyte Changes in HIV-Infected Mothers and Their Infants*. IVth International Conference on AIDS, Stockholm, Sweden (1988).

56. Rubinstein, E., Madden, G., Smith, C., Lyons, R., *Improved Survival from Time of AIDS Diagnosis for Intravenous Drug Users Diagnosed in 1987*. VIth International Conference on AIDS, San Francisco, CA (1990).

57. Sugland, B., Hidalgo, J., Chaisson, R., Moore, R., *Impact of Zidovudine and Other Factors on the Natural History of AIDS*. VIth International Conference on AIDS, San Francisco, CA (1990).

58. Volberding, P., Lagakos, S., Koch, M., et al, *Zidovudine Therapy of Asymptomatic HIV Infected Persons with Less than 500 CD4+ Cells/mm3-ACTG Protocol 019*. VIth International Conference on AIDS, San Francisco, CA (1990).

59. Seage, G., Oddleifson, S., Carr, E., et al, *Survival with AIDS in Massachusetts, 1981-1988*. VIth International Conference on AIDS, San Francisco, CA (1990).

60. Payne, S., Lemp, G., Franks, D., Rutherford, G., *Survival Following Diagnosis of AIDS-Related Opportunistic Infections in San Francisco*. VIth International Conference on AIDS, San Francisco, CA (1990).

61. Lafferty, W., Glidden, D., Hopkins, S., et al, *Increased Survival for PWA*. Vth International Conference on AIDS, Montreal, Canada (1989).

62. Haley, C., Reffe, Fifth., Freeman, A., Haslund, I., et al, *Improved Survival of AIDS Patients in Dallas, Texas After 1986*. Vth International Conference on AIDS, Montreal, Canada (1989).

63. Earl, W., Martindale, C., Cohn, D., *Denial: The Continuum of Coping Mechanism Styles with Regard to HIV Infection*. VIth International Conference on AIDS, San Francisco, CA (1990).

64. Ostrow, D., Beltran, E., Wesch, J., Joseph, J., *Recreational Drug Use and Homosexual Behavior: The Role of Volatile Nitrites ("Poppers") in Explaining the Association*. VIth International Conference on AIDS, San Francisco, CA (1990).

65. Moulton, J., Stempel, R., Bacchetti, P., et al, *Results of a Longitudinal Psychosocial Study of the Impact of Antibody Test Notification*. IVth International Conference on AIDS, Stockholm, Sweden (1988).

66. Rodriguez, R., Herbert, M., Kemeny, M., et al, *A Comparison of Coping Responses Between Gay Men Who Know and Do Not Know Their HIV Status*. VIth International Conference on AIDS, San Francisco, CA (1990).

67. Casadonte, P., DesJarlais, D., Friedman, S., et al, *Psychological & Behavioral Impact of Learning HIV Test Results in I.V. Drug Users*. IVth International Conference on AIDS, Stockholm, Sweden (1988).

68. Satz, P., Miller, E., Visscher, B., et al, *Changes in Mood as a Function of HIV Serostatus: A 3-Year Longitudinal Study*. IVth International Conference on AIDS, Stockholm, Sweden (1988).

69. Green, T., Karon, J., Stehr-Green, J., *Changes in U.S. AIDS Incidence Trends*. CDC, Atlanta, GA, VIth International Conference on AIDS, San Francisco, CA (1990).

70. Coates, Thomas J., Morin, S., McKusick, L., et al, *Long-Term Consequences of AIDS Antibody Testing on Gay and Bisexual Men.* IVth International Conference on AIDS, Stockholm, Sweden (1988).

71. *Hemophilia Information Exchange.* AIDS UPDATE, Chapter Advisory #86, Medical Bulletin #76, The National Hemophilia Foundation, NY, NY, 2/14/89.

72. Killinger, J., Kroner, B., White, G., et al, *Safe Sex Practices of Female Partners of Hemophilic Men.* VIth International Conference on AIDS, San Francisco, CA (1990).

73. Ekstrand, M., Coates, T., Lang, S., Guydish, J., *Prevalence and Change of AIDS High Risk Sexual Behavior Among Bisexual Men in San Francisco: The San Francisco Men's Health Study.* Vth International Conference on AIDS, Montreal, Canada (1989).

74. Strawn, J., *AIDS Health Attitude Survey.* VIth International Conference on AIDS, San Francisco, CA (1990).

75. Wallston, B., Alagna, S., DeVellis, B., DeVellis, R., Social Support and Physical Health. *Health Psychology,* 2, 367–391. (1983).

76. Dorus, W., Schaefer, M., Lention, J., et al, *IVDU'S Psychological, Behavioral, Attitudinal Status and Level of Knowledge About HIV After HIV Testing and Education.* VIth International Conference on AIDS, San Francisco, CA (1990).

77. Farley, T., Carter, M., Hadler, J., *HIV Counseling and Testing in Methadone Programs: Effect on Treatment Compliance.* VIth International Conference on AIDS, San Francisco, CA (1990).

78. Patel, R., Brandon, D., Altman, R., Robeson, L., Pizzuti, W., *HIV-1 Infection Among Non-IVDU's Admitted to Drug Treatment Programs.* VIth International Conference on AIDS, San Francisco, CA (1990).

79. Calsyn, D., Saxon, A., Freeman, Jr., *Correlates of HIV Risk Reduction Among IVDU's.* VIth International Conference on AIDS, San Francisco, CA (1990).

80. Holman, S., Sunderland, A., Moroso, G., et al, *Multidisciplinary Model for HIV Testing of Pregnant Women in a Drug Treatment Program.* IVth International Conference on AIDS, Stockholm, Sweden (1988).

81. MacGregor, R.R., "Alcohol and Immune Defense." *JAMA,* 256: 1474–1479. (1986).

82. Jerrells, T., Marietta, A., Bone, G., Weight, F., Eckardt, M., *Ethanol-Associated Immunosuppression. Psychological, Neuropsychiatric, and Substance Abuse Aspects of AIDS. Advances in Biochemical Psychopharmacology,* vol. 44; 173–185, Raven Press, (1988).

83. Friedman, H., Klein, T., Specter, S., Pross, S., et al, *Drugs of Abuse and Virus Susceptibility. Psychological, Neuropsychiatric, and Substance Abuse Aspects of AIDS. Advances in Biochemical Psychopharmacology,* vol. 44, 125–137, Raven Press, (1988).

84. Naber, D., Perro, D., Schick, Einhaupl, K., *Psychiatric Symptoms and Neuro-psychological Functioning in HIV-Infected Patients. Etiology?* VIth International Conference on AIDS, San Francisco, CA (1990).

85. Marder, K., Malouf, R., Doonelef, G., et al, *Neurological Signs and Symptoms in Parenteral Drug Users.* VIth International Conference on AIDS, San Francisco, CA (1990).

86. Nichols, S., Ostrow, D., *Clinical Insights: Psychiatric Implications of Acquired Immune Deficiency Syndrome.* American Psychiatric Association, 1984.

87. Chuang, H., Jason, G., Pajurkova, E., Gill, M., *Psychiatric Morbidity In HIV Infection.* VIth International Conference on AIDS, San Francisco, CA (1990).

88. Lai, P., Takayama, H., Tamura, Y., Nonoyama, M., *Activation of Human Immunodeficiency Virus in Human Myeloid Cells by Cocaine.* VIth International Conference on AIDS, San Francisco, CA (1990).

89. Chiasson, M.A., Stoneburner, R., Hildebrandt, D., et al, *Heterosexual Transmission of HIV Associated with the Use of Smokable Freebase Cocaine (Crack).* VIth International Conference on AIDS, San Francisco, CA (1990).

90. Nenoto, T., Brown, L., Battjes, R., Siddiqui, N., *Patterns of Cocaine Use in Relation to HIV Infection Among Intravenous Drug Users in New York City.* VIth International Conference on AIDS, San Francisco, CA (1990).

91. Amsel, Z., Battjes, R., Pickens, R., *Cocaine Use and HIV Risk Among Intravenous Opiate Addicts.* VIth International Conference on AIDS, San Francisco, CA (1990).

92. Schoenbaum, E., Hartel, D., Friedland, G., *Crack Use Predicts Incident HIV Seroconversion.* VIth International Conference on AIDS, San Francisco, CA (1990).

93. Weissman, G., Sowder, B., Young, P., *The Relationship Between Crack Cocaine Use and Other Risk Factors Among Women in a National AIDS Prevention Program—U.S., Puerto Rico and Mexico.* VIth International Conference on AIDS, San Francisco, CA (1990).

94. Wiebel, W., Guydan, C., Chene, D., *Cocaine Injection as a Predictor of HIV Risk Behaviors.* VIth International Conference on AIDS, San Francisco, CA (1990).

95. Ostrow, D., Beltran, E., Wesch, J., Joseph, J., *Recreational Drug Use and Homosexual Behavior: The Role of Volatile Nitrites ("Poppers") In Explaining the Association.* VIth International Conference on AIDS, San Francisco, CA (1990).

96. Seage, G., Third, Mayer, K., Horsburgh, C., Holmberg, S., Lamb, G., *Evaluation of the Role of Nitrite Inhalents in HIV Transmission: Confounding or Effect Modifications?* Vth International Conference on AIDS, Montreal, Canada (1989).

97. O'Reilly, K., Higgins, D., Galavotti, C., Sheridan, J., *Relapse from Safer Sex Among Homosexual Men: Evidence from Four Cohorts in the AIDS Community Demonstration Projects.* CDC, Atlanta, GA, VIth International Conference on AIDS, San Francisco, CA (1990).

98. Harris, N., Schlberg, E., Livingston, G., *HIV Spread Among Intravenous Drug Users (IVDUs) in King County, Washington.* VIth International Conference on AIDS, San Francisco, CA (1990).

99. Bartholow, B., Cohn, D., Cole, V., et al, *From Low-Risk to High-Risk: Distinguishing Among Groups of Gay Men on the HIV Risk Relapse Continuum.* CDC, Atlanta, GA, VIth International Conference on AIDS, San Francisco, CA (1990).

100. St. Lawrence, J., Brasfield, T., Kelly, J., *Factors Which Predict Relapse to Unsafe Sex by Gay Men.* VIth International Conference on AIDS, San Francisco, CA (1990).

101. Morris, R., Re, O., Baker, C., et al, *Survey of Sexually Transmitted Diseases and Drug Abuse Risk Factors for HIV Infection in Incarcerated Adolescents.* VIth International Conference on AIDS, San Francisco, CA (1990).

102. Haignere, C., Rotheram-Borus, J., Koopman, et al, *HIV/AIDS Prevention and Multiple Risk Behaviors of Gay Male and Runaway Adolescents.* VIth International Conference on AIDS, San Francisco, CA (1990).

103. McKusick, L., Coates, T., Stall, R., et al, *Psychosocial and Behavioral Predictors of AIDS Risk Reduction.* IVth International Conference on AIDS, Stockholm, Sweden (1988).

104. Hartel, D., Selwyn, P., Schoenbaum, E.E., et al, *Methadone Maintenance Treatment (MMTP) and Reduced Risk of AIDS and AIDS-Specific Mortality in Intravenous Drug Users (IVDUs).* IVth International Conference on AIDS, Stockholm, Sweden (1988).

105. Blix, O., Grönbladh, L., *AIDS and Fourth Heroin Addicts: The Preventive Effect of Methadone Maintenance in Sweden.* IVth International Conference on AIDS, Stockholm, Sweden (1988).

106. Remien, R., Rabkin, J., Williams, J., Gorman, J., Ehrhardt, A., *Cessation of Alcohol and Drug Use Disorders in an HIV Sample.* Vth International Conference on AIDS, Montreal, Canada (1989).

107. Arora, P., Fride, E., Petitto, J., et al, *Morphine-Induced Modulation of the Immune System: Implications for AIDS.* IVth International Conference on AIDS, Stockholm, Sweden (1988).

108. Klimas, N., Page, B., Chitwood, D., et al, *Immune Abnormalities in Street Intravenous Drug Users.* IVth International Conference on AIDS, Stockholm, Sweden (1988).

109. Mientzes, G., van den Hoek, JAR, van Ameijden, E., et al, *The Impact of Frequent Injecting on the Immune Status of Intravenous Drug Users.* VIth International Conference on AIDS, San Francisco, CA (1990).

110. Blaney, N.T., Klimas, N.G., Fletcher, M.A., *Mood State, Social Support and Immune Function in HIV− and HIV+ I.V. Drug Abusers, an AIDS Risk Group.* IVth International Conference on AIDS, Stockholm, Sweden (1988).

111. Magura, S., Herman, J., Rosenblum, A., Feffers, J., et al, *Reducing HIV Transmission by Providing Methadone Treatment to Intravenous Drug Users in Jail.* Vth International Conference on AIDS, Montreal, Canada (1989).

112. Williams, A., Vranizan, K., Gorter, R., et al, *Methadone Maintenance, HIV Serostatus and Race in Injection Drug Users in San Francisco, CA.* VIth International Conference on AIDS, San Francisco, CA (1990).

113. Bagasra, O., Lischner, H., Kajdacsy-Balla, A., *Increased Susceptibility of Unstimulated Peripheral Blood Mononuclear Cells (PBMC) and CD8+ Cell-Depleted PBMC to In Vitro Infection with HIV after Ingestion of 2–4 Beers.* Vth International Conference on AIDS, Montreal, Canada (1989).

114. Rosenberger, P., Bornstein, R., Nasrallah, et al; *Psychiatric Disorder in HIV Infected Gay Males.* VIth International Conference on AIDS, San Francisco, CA (1990).

115. Finnegan, D., McNalley, E., *Dual Identities.* 1987, 31–32, Hazelden, USA.

116. Saghir, M., Robins, E., Walbran, B., Gentry, K., "Homosexuality: Third. Psychiatric Disorders and Disability in the Male Homosexual." *American Journal of Psychiatry,* 126(8) 1970a, 1079–1086.

117. Saghir, M., Robins, E., Walbran, B., Gentry, K., "Homosexuality: Fourth. Psychiatric Disorders and Disability in the Female Homosexual." *American Journal of Psychiatry,* 127(2) 1970b, 147–154.

118. Lohrenz, L., Connely, J., Coyne, L., Spare, K., "Alcohol Problems in Several Midwestern Homosexual Communities." *Journal of Studies on Alcohol,* 39, 1959–1963.

119. Peterson, P., McKirnan, D., *Gay Identification Influences the Effects of Alcohol Use on AIDS Risk Behavior.* Vth International Conference on AIDS, Montreal, Canada (1989).

120. Yano, E., Gorman, E., Kanouse, D., et al, *The Epidemiology of Risk Behavior in Los Angeles: Population-Based Comparison of Gay/Bisexual Men and the General Population.* VIth International Conference on AIDS, San Francisco, CA (1990).

121. Ferguson, M., "Group Therapy Support Increases Cancer Survival." *Brain Mind Bulletin,* 14:11, 1–6, Interface Press (August 1989).

122. Jacobs, J., Ilaria, G., *Management of Psychological Distress: A Hospital Based "Mutual AID" Support Group for HIV Seropositive Men.* Center for Special Studies, New York Hospital-Cornell Medical Center, N.Y., N.Y.

123. Kelly, J., Lawrence, J., *The AIDS Health Crisis: Psychological and Social Interventions.* 93–117, Plenum Press, N.Y. (1988).

124. Gandil, P., Andersen, T., Bjorner, J., *A Model for Psycho-Social Support and Counselling.* VIth International Conference on AIDS, San Francisco, CA (1990).

125. Karl, S., Eck, E., *Living Healthy with HIV.* VIth International Conference on AIDS, San Francisco, CA (1990).

126. Fleishman, J., Piette, J., Mor, V., *Correlates of Depressive Symptomatology Among People with AIDS.* VIth International Conference on AIDS, San Francisco, CA (1990).

127. Eric, K., Druckar, E., Worth, D., Chabon, D., et al, *The Women's Center: A Model Peer Support Program for High Risk Fourth Drug and Crack Using Women in the Bronx.* Vth International Conference on AIDS, Montreal, Canada (1989).

128. Balthazar, H., *Self Help Groups and the AIDS Patients.* Vth International Conference on AIDS, Montreal, Canada (1989).

129. Friedman, S., Serrano, Y., Torres, L., Sufian, M., et al, *Organizing Intravenous Drug Users Against AIDS.* Vth International Conference on AIDS, Montreal, Canada (1989).

130. Freeman, Anne C., Anderson, P., Reff, Fifth., *Use of Facilitated Peer Support*

Group to Effect Behavior Change in HIV Positive Individuals. IVth International Conference on AIDS, Stockholm, Sweden (1988).

131. Baker, Peter, Helbert, Matthew, *Self Help Groups for People With AIDS.* IVth International Conference on AIDS, Stockholm, Sweden (1988).

132. Reillo, M., *Psychosocial Factors Associated with Prognosis in AIDS.* VIth International Conference on AIDS, San Francisco, CA (1990).

133. Barret, R., Robinson, B., *Reducing Unsafe Sexual Practices of HIV Seropositive Gay Men: Education, Counseling, and the Twelve Steps.* IVth International Conference on AIDS, Stockholm, Sweden (1988).

134. Melton, G., *Beyond AIDS. A Journey Into Healing.* Brotherhood Press, Beverly Hills, CA, 1988.

135. Pennebaker, J., Kiecolt-Glaser, J., Glaser, R., "Disclosure of traumas and immune function: Health implications for Psychotherapy." *Journal of Consulting and Clinical Psychology,* vol. 56, No. 2, 239–245, 1989.

CHAPTER TWO REFERENCES

1. Temoshok, L., O'Leary, A., Jenkins, S., Henry, M., *Survival Time in Men with AIDS: Relationships with Psychological Coping and Autonomic Arousal.* VIth International Conference on AIDS, San Francisco, CA, 1990.

2. Lawrence, Dale N., Jason, J.M., Holman, R.C., et al, *Heterosexual Transmission of HIV-Infected U.S. Hemophilic Men.* Centers for Disease Control, Atlanta, GA, IVth International Conference on AIDS, Stockholm, Sweden (1988).

3. Robertson, K., Wilkins, J., Bowdre, J., et al, *Psychological Influences on Herpes Simplex Virus Titers in HIV+ Subjects.* VIth International Conference on AIDS, San Francisco, CA (1990).

4. Ellis, A., McInerney, J., DiGiuseppe, R., Yeager, R., *Rational-Emotive Therapy with Alcoholics and Substance Abusers.* Pergamon Press, Elmsford, New York, 1988.

5. Kobasa, S., Maddi, S., Kahn, S., "Hardiness and Health: a Prospective Study." *Journal of Personality and Social Psychology.* 42:168–177, 1982.

6. Kobasa, S., Maddi, S., Puccetti, M., "Personality and Exercise as Buffers in the Stress-Illness Relationship." *Journal of Behavioral Medicine.* 4:391–404, 1982.

7. Mellody, P., *Facing Codependence.* Harper and Row, San Francisco, CA, 1989.

CHAPTER THREE REFERENCES

1. Frankl, Viktor, *Man's Search for Meaning. An Introduction to Logotherapy.* Washington Square Press, New York, New York, 1963.

2. Laperriere, A., Ironson, G., O'Hearn, P., et al, *Aerobic Exercise Training as a Buffer of Anxiety and Depression in HIV Infected Individuals.* Poster to Society of Behavioral Medicine, San Francisco, CA, 1989.

CHAPTER FIFTEEN:
HEALTH CARE PROVIDERS REFERENCES

1. DeMayo, M., Miller, R., *Reinforcing Safer Sex and Preventing Relapse to High-Risk Behaviors Among Gay Men.* VIth International Conference on AIDS, San Francisco, CA (1990).

2. Felch, F., Fitzgerald, B., LaChapelis, R., Santiago, V., *Combined AIDS and Addiction Service Delivery in an Anonymous Drop-In HIV Test Site—Project TRUST.* VIth International Conference on AIDS, San Francisco, CA (1990).

3. Atkinson, H., Gutierrez, R., Cottler, L., et al, *Suicide Ideation and Attempts in HIV Illness.* VIth International Conference on AIDS, San Francisco, CA (1990).

4. Nichols, S., Ostrow, D., *Clinical Insights: Psychiatric Implications of Acquired Immune Deficiency Syndrome.* American Psychiatric Association, 1984.

5. Barret, Robert L., Robinson, Bryan E., *Reducing Unsafe Sexual Practices of HIV Seropositive Gay Men: Education, Counseling and the Twelve Steps.* IVth International Conference on AIDS, Stockholm, Sweden (1988).

6. *People with AIDS: Partners in the Provision of Services.* National Association of People with AIDS. IVth International Conference on AIDS, Stockholm, Sweden (1988).

7. Pivar, I., Temoshok, L., *Coping Strategies and Response Styles in Homosexual Symptomatic Seropositive Men.* VIth International Conference on AIDS, San Francisco, CA, (1990).

8. Reed, G., Kemeny, M., Taylor, S., *Coping Responses and Psychological Adjustment in Gay Men with AIDS: A Longitudinal Analysis.* VIth International Conference on AIDS, San Francisco, CA (1990).

9. Kelly, B., Raphael, B., Zournazi, A., Dunne, M., Smith, S., *Psychological Adjustment to HIV Infection.* VIth International Conference on AIDS, San Francisco, CA (1990).

10. Phillips, C., Folkman, S., Pollack, L., Chesney, M., *Not Stress, But How You Cope With It Is Related to Sexual Risk Behavior Among Gay Men.* VIth International Conference on AIDS, San Francisco, CA (1990).

11. Storosum, I., Van den Boom, F., Van Beuzekom, M., Sno, H., *Stress and Coping in People with HIV-Infection.* VIth International Conference on AIDS, San Francisco, CA (1990).

12. Greer, S., Watson, M., "Mental adjustment to cancer: Its management and prognostic significance." *Cancer Surveys*, 6, 439–454, 1987.

13. Pettingale, K., Morris, T., Greer, S., Haybittle, J., "Mental attitudes to cancer: an additional prognostic factor." *Lancet* I:750, 1985.38.

14. Temoshok, L., Heller, B., Sagebiel, R., et al, "The relationship of psychosocial factors to prognostic indicators in cutaneous malignant melanoma." *Journal of Psychosomatic Research*, 29:139–153, 1985.

15. Temoshok, L., "Personality, coping style, emotion, and cancer: Toward an integrative model." *Cancer Surveys*, 6, 545–568, 1987.

16. Stolbach, L., Brandt, U., "Psychosocial factors in the development and progression of breast cancer." *Stress and Breast Cancer*. Cooper, C., (Eds.) John Wiley & Sons, Ltd, 1988.

17. Long, D., Hodel, D., Meally, R., et al, *The Necessity of Self-Empowerment by the Person with HIV*. VIth International Conference on AIDS, San Francisco, CA (1990).

18. Marchand-Gonod, N., Edel, Y., Rodriguez, J., Gentilini, M., *Incidence of Depression Among 30 Homosexual Men with Clinical AIDS Hospitalized over an 18 Month Period*. VIth International Conference on AIDS, San Francisco, CA (1990).

19. Hedge, B., Green, J., *Evaluation of Focused Cognitive-Behavioral Intervention with HIV Seropositive Individuals*. VIth International Conference on AIDS, San Francisco, CA (1990).

20. Krell, P., Winsiewski, A., Jensen, P., *Relationship between Cognitive Dysfunction and Mood State at Different Stages of HIV Disease*. VIth International Conference on AIDS, San Francisco, CA (1990).

21. Gutierrez, R., Atkinson, H., Velin, R., et al, *Coping and Neuropsychological Correlates of Suicidality in HIV*. VIth International Conference on AIDS, San Francisco, CA (1990).

22. Keller, S., Bartlett, J., Schleifer, S., et al, *Human Immunodeficiency Virus Infection and HIV-Relevant Sexual Behavior among a Healthy Inner-City Heterosexual Adolescent Population*. VIth IInternational Conference on AIDS, San Francisco, CA (1990).

23. Canick, J., Temoshok, L., *The Longitudinal Assessment of Perceived and Objective Cognitive Impairment in Symptomatic HIV Seropositive Men*. VIth International Conference on AIDS, San Francisco, CA (1990).

24. Nyamathi, A., Flaskerud, J., *Effect of Coherence, Self Esteem and Support-Available as Resources Against Emotional and Physical Distress and High Risk Behaviors in Minority Women*. VIth International Conference on AIDS, San Francisco, CA (1990).

25. Tunstall, C., Cooper, F., Oliva, G., et al, *Addressing Psychological Barriers to the Prevention of HIV Infection in High-Risk Women*. VIth International Conference on AIDS, San Francisco, CA (1990).

26. Grace, W., Rundell, J., Oster, C., *Types of Social Support and Their Relationships to Depressive Symptoms in HIV Positive Men*. VIth International Conference on AIDS, San Francisco, CA (1990).

27. Zierler, S., Feingold, L., Laufer, D., et al, *Risk of Adult HIV Infection and Childhood Sexual Abuse*. Vth International Conference on AIDS, Montreal, Canada (1989).

28. Coates, T., McKusick, L., *The Efficacy of Stress Management in Reducing High Risk Behavior and Improving Immune Function in HIV Antibody Positive Men.* IIIrd International Conference on AIDS, Washington, D.C. (1987).

29. Kelly, J., Lawrence, J., *The AIDS Health Crisis: Psychological and Social Interventions.* 93–117, Plenum Press, N.Y., 1988.

30. Antoni, M., Fletcher, M., Laperriere, A., et al, *Stress Management, Psychological and Immune Functioning among Asymptomatic HIV+ and HIV− Gay Males.* Scientific Meetings of the American Association for the Advancement of Science, San Francisco, CA, 1989.

31. Collinge, W., Lessa-Zielinski, D., *HIV and Quality of Life: Outcomes of a Psychosocial Intervention Program.* Poster to Society of Behavioral Medicine, San Francisco, CA, 1989.

32. Antoni, H., August, S., Baggett, H., et al, *Stress Management as Buffer of Anxiety Increments and Immunologic Decrements During Five-Week Period Preceding HIV-1 Serostatus Notification.* VIth International Conference on AIDS, San Francisco, CA (1990).

33. Kiecolt-Glaser, J., Glaser, R., Williger, D., et al, "Psychosocial Enhancement of Immunocompetence in a Geriatric Population." *Health Psychology,* 4(1), 25–41, 1985.

34. Kiecolt-Glaser, J., Glaser, R., Strain, E., et al, Modulation of Cellular Immunity in Medical Students. *Journal of Behavioral Medicine,* 9, 311–320, 1986.

35. Baggett, H., Antoni, M., et al, *Frequency of Relaxation Practice, State Anxiety, and Immune Markers in an HIV-1 High Risk Group.* Poster to Society of Behavioral Medicine, San Francisco, CA, 1989.

36. Valdimarsdottir, H., Stone, A., Cox, D., Neale, J., *Relaxation and Experimental Stressors affect Interleukin-2 and Lymphocyte Proliferation.* Poster to Society of Behavioral Medicine, San Francisco, CA, 1989.

37. Gruber, B., Hall, N., Hersh, S., *Immune System Changes in Breast Cancer Patients Given Relaxation, Guided Imagery and Biofeedback Training.* Paper to Association for Applied Psychophysiology and Biofeedback, San Diego, 1989.

38. Ladd, C., Schumann-Brezezinski, D., McGrady, S., Conran, P., *Effect of Biofeedback Assisted Relaxation on Cellular Immunity.* Poster to Association for Applied Psychophysiology and Biofeedback, San Diego, CA (1989).

39. Hamilton, B., Dufault, E., *The Use of Three Biopsychosocial Interventions of the Stress Levels and Immune Functioning of HIV Positive Individuals.* Vth International Conference on AIDS, Montreal, Canada (1989).

40. Ironson, G., Laperriere, A., August, S., et al, *Correlations of Immune Function with Mood and Coping Measures Over Time in an AIDS Risk Group.* Poster to Society of Behavioral Medicine, San Francisco, CA, 1989.

41. Goldstein, D., Antoni, M., Llabre, M., et al, *Repressive Coping Style is Associated with Tumor Size and Clinical Stage in Breast Cancer.* Poster to Society of Behavioral Medicine, San Francisco, CA, 1989.

42. Wolf, T., Dralle, P., Morse, E., et al, *The HIV-Infected Patient and Family*

Social Support. Poster presented to the Society of Behavioral Medicine, San Francisco, CA, 1989.

43. Brown, S., O'Leary, A., *Psychosocial Correlates of Immune Function in a Healthy Elderly Cohort*. Poster to Society of Behavioral Medicine, San Francisco, CA, 1989.

44. Namir, S., Wolcott, D., Fawzy, F., Alumbaugh, M., "Coping with AIDS: Psychological and Health Implications." *Journal of Applied Social Psychology,* 17, (3), 309–328, 1987.

45. Temoshok, L., Stites, D.P., Sweet, D.M., et al, *A Psychoimmunologic Study of Men with ARC.* IVth International Conference on AIDS, Stockholm, Sweden (1988).

46. Millon, C., Morgan, R., Blaney, N., et al, *Personality Style, Psychosocial Variables and Immune Status in an HIV Positive Population*. IVth International Conference on AIDS, Stockholm, Sweden (1988).

47. Baum, A., and Temoshok, L., (Eds.), *Psychological Aspects of AIDS*. Hillsdale, N.Y.: Lawrence Erlbaum Associates, Inc. (1989).

48. August, S., Ironson, G., Laperriere, A., et al, *Notification of HIV-1 Antibody Status: Coping and Mood State in Healthy Gay Men*. Poster to Society of Behavioral Medicine, San Francisco, CA, 1989.

49. Blaney, N.T., Klimas, N.G., Fletcher, M.A., *Mood State, Social Support and Immune Function in HIV− and HIV+ IV Drug Abusers, an AIDS Risk Group*. IVth International Conference on AIDS, Stockholm, Sweden (1988).

50. McKusick, Leon, Coates, T.J., Morin, S., *Self Efficacy and Community Norms Predict AIDS Risk Reduction Among Gay and Bisexual Men in San Francisco: The AIDS Behavioral Research Project*. Vth International Conference on AIDS, Montreal, Canada (1989).

51. Kelly, P., *Evaluation of a Meditation and Hypnosis-Based Stress Management Program for Men with HIV*. Vth International Conference on AIDS, Montreal, Canada (1989).

52. Kemeny, M., Duran, R., Taylor, S., et al, *Chronic Depression Predicts CD4 Decline Over a Five Year Period in HIV Seropositive Men*. VIth International Conference on AIDS, San Francisco, CA (1990).

53. Mehl, L., Chan, B., *Possible Placebo Effect in AIDS and ARC*. VIth International Conference on AIDS, San Francisco, CA (1990).

54. Schmidt, M., McKirnan, D., Tramner, P., *Social, Emotional, and Neuropsychological Components of Functional Status in Minority AIDS Patients*. VIth International Conference on AIDS, San Francisco, CA (1990).

55. Turner, H., Hays, R., Coates, T., *Determinants of Social Support Among Gay Men*. VIth International Conference on AIDS, San Francisco, CA (1990).

56. Earl, W., Flinders, R., Flahive, M., et al, *Psychosocial Adjustment to HIV Infection: Efficacy of Different Group Interventions in Gay and Bisexual Men*. VIth International Conference on AIDS, San Francisco, CA (1990).

57. Freeman, M., *Therapeutic Narrative: Multi-Media Uses of Cross-Cultural Storytelling for People Living with AIDS*. VIth International Conference on AIDS, San Francisco, CA (1990).

References

58. Ingram, F., Laperriere, A., Antoni, M., et al, *Effects of a Behavioral Intervention on Coping Behaviors in Healthy Males at Risk for AIDS*. Poster to Society of Behavioral Medicine, San Francisco, CA, 1989.

59. Temoshok, L., Canick, J., Moulton, J.M., et al, *Distress, Coping, and Neuropsychological Status in Men with ARC: Longitudinal Studies*. IVth International Conference on AIDS, Stockholm, Sweden (1988).

60. Laperriere, A., Ironson, G., O'Hearn, P., et al, *Aerobic Exercise Training as a Buffer of Anxiety and Depression in HIV Infected Individuals*. Poster to Society of Behavioral Medicine, San Francisco, CA, 1989.

61. Ingram, F., Laperriere, A., Ironson, G., et al, *Influence of Loneliness and Social Support on the Effectiveness of a Behavioral Intervention with Healthy Males at Risk for AIDS*. Vth International Conference on AIDS, Montreal, Canada (1989).

62. Baker, P., Helbert, M., *Self Help Groups for People With AIDS*. IVth International Conference on AIDS, Stockholm, Sweden (1988).

63. Freeman, A., Anderson, P., Reff, Fifth., *Use of Facilitated Peer Support Group to Effect Behavior Change in HIV Positive Individuals*. IVth International Conference on AIDS, Stockholm, Sweden (1988).

64. Solomon, K., Rosenthal, S., James, R., et al, *HIV Positive Support Groups—A Model of Intervention*. Vth International Conference on AIDS, Montreal, Canada (1989).

65. Schilling, R., El-Bassel, N., Gordon, K., et al, *Reducing HIV Transmission Among Recovering Female Drug Users*. Vth International Conference on AIDS, Montreal, Canada (1989).

66. Magura, S., Shapiro, J.L., Siddiqui, Q., et al, *Variables Influencing Condom Use Among Intravenous Drug Users*. Vth International Conference on AIDS, Montreal, Canada (1989).

67. DiClemente, R., DuNah, R., *Influence of Perceived Referent-Group Normative Behavior on Adolescents Use of Condoms*. Vth International Conference on AIDS, Montreal, Canada (1989).

68. Hays, R., Turner, H., Catania, J., et al, *Social Support, HIV Symptoms and Depression Among Gay Men*. Vth International Conference on AIDS, Montreal, Canada (1989).

69. Jacobs, J., Miller, S., Streeter, N., *Comprehensive Volunteer Program for People with AIDS*. Vth International Conference on AIDS, Montreal, Canada (1989).

70. Pelfini, A., *Integrated Identity Through the Emotional Support Approach*. Vth International Conference on AIDS, Montreal, Canada (1989).

71. Hayes, R., Catania, J., McKusick, L., Coates, T., *Help-Seeking for AIDS-related Concerns: A Comparison of Gay Men with Various HIV Diagnoses*. Vth International Conference on AIDS, Montreal, Canada (1989).

72. Arnold, W., Barnes, F., *Peer Education Program Reaches High Risk Adolescents with AIDS Information and Prevention*. Vth International Conference on AIDS, Montreal, Canada (1989).

73. Greenblatt, R., Catania, J., Kegeles, S., Schachter, J., Miller, J., Coates, T., et al, *Predictors of Condom Use and STDs in a Group of Sexually Active Adolescent Women*. Vth International Conference on AIDS, Montreal, Canada (1989).

74. Hayman, C., Peterson, L., Miller, C., *HIV Infection in Underprivileged Teen-agers Update from the Job Corps*. VIth International Conference on AIDS, San Francisco, CA (1990).

75. Rotheram-Borus, J., Koopman, C., Haignere, C., et al, *An Effective Program for Changing Sexual Risk Behaviors of Gay Male and Runaway Adolescents*. VIth International Conference on AIDS, San Francisco, CA (1990).

76. Cassel, J., *Am. J. Edpdemiol*. 104, 107 (1976).

77. Cobb, S., *Psychosomatic Med*. 38, 300 (1976).

78. Cohen, S., Syme, S., *Social Support and Health*. Academic Press, New York, 1985.

79. Cassileth, B., Walsh, W., Lusk, E., "Psychosocial Correlates of Cancer Survival: A Subsequent Report 3 to 8 Years after Cancer Diagnosis." *Journal of Clinical Oncology*, 6, 11, 1753–1759, 1988.

80. House, J., et al, "Social relationships and health." *Science*, 241, 540–545, July 29, 1988.

81. Piersigilli, R., Speranza, T., Salis, P., et al, *Burnout in Health Care Workers Caring PWA*. VIth International Conference on AIDS, San Francisco, CA (1990).

82. Healy-Chidekel, J., Patrone-Reese, J., Almunia, M., et al, *The University of Miami/AIDS Clinical Research Unit: A Model Program which Facilitates Staff Retention and Decreases "Burnout" for AIDS Health Care Providers*. VIth International Conference on AIDS, San Francisco, CA (1990).

83. Raveis, V., Siegel, K., Kletecka, C., et al, *Adequacy of Informal Support to Gay Men with AIDS and the Psychosocial Consequences for the Caregiver*. VIth International Conference on AIDS, San Francisco, CA (1990).

84. Cadwell, S., *Issues of Identification for Gay Psychotherapists Treating Gay Clients with HIV Spectrum Disorder: Special Vulnerability and its Management*. VIth International Conference on AIDS, San Francisco, CA (1990).

RESOURCES APPENDIX

Addictions Recovery

TWELVE STEP SUPPORT GROUPS NATIONAL NUMBERS
(check local listings in white pages—local AA central offices will list special groups, i.e. gay/lesbian and HIV+)

Alcoholics Anonymous World Services, Inc.
  Box 459, Grand Central Station, New York, NY 10017
  (212) 686-1100

Al-Anon Family Groups
  P.O. Box 862, Midtown Station, New York, NY 10018
  (212) 302-7240

Adult Children of Alcoholics
  2522 W. Sepulveda Blvd., Torrance, CA 90505
  (213) 534-1815

Assessment Center (24-hour alcohol and drug abuse referral line)
  (800) 852-5209

Co-Dependents Anonymous
  P.O. Box 33577, Phoenix, AZ 85067-3577
  (602) 277-7991

Codependents of Sex Addicts
  P.O. Box 14537, Minneapolis, MN 55414
  (612) 537-6904

Narcotics Anonymous
  World Service Office, P.O. Box 9999, Van Nuys, CA 91409
  (818) 780-3951

Sexaholics Anonymous (SA), International Central Office
  P.O. Box 300, Simi Valley, CA 93062
  (805) 581-3343

S-Anon International Family Groups
  P.O. Box 5117, Sherman Oaks, CA 91413
  (818) 990-6910

Sex and Love Addicts Anonymous (S.L.A.A.)
4391 Sunset Blvd., #520, Los Angeles, CA 90029
(213) 859-5585

Sexual Addicts Anonymous (SAA)
P.O. Box 3038, Minneapolis, MN 55403
(612) 871-1520

Sexual Compulsives Anonymous
P.O. Box 1585, Old Chelsea Station, New York, NY 10011
(212) 439-1123

ADDICTION HOTLINES

Alcohol Abuse and Assistance Helpline and Hospital Referral for
Alcohol, Drug and Cocaine Addiction
(800) 333-4444
National Institute on Drug Abuse Hotline
(800) 662-HELP (662-4357)
National Council on Alcoholism and Drug Dependence
(800) 475-HOPE (475-4673)

ADDICTION ORGANIZATIONS / CENTERS

American Society of Addiction Medicine, Inc.
12 West 21st St., New York, NY 10010
(212) 206-6770
5225 Wisconsin Ave., N.W., Suite 409, Washington, D.C. 20015
(202) 244-8948

Pride Institute (substance abuse treatment for gays and lesbians)
14400 Martin Dr., Eden Prairie, MN 55344
(800) 54-PRIDE (547-7433)

National Association of Lesbian and Gay Alcoholism Professionals
204 W. 20th St., New York, NY 10011
(212) 713-5074

National Clearinghouse for Alcohol & Drug Information
Box 2345, Rockville, MD 20852
(301) 468-2600

National Self-Help Clearinghouse
25 W. 43rd St., Room 620, New York, NY 10036

Recovery Alliance (people recovering from addictions with HIV-AIDS and health professionals)
2025 Nicollet Ave., Minneapolis, MN 55404
(612) 870-7773

AIDS/HIV Infection

HOTLINES

AIDS Clinical Trials Information Service
(800) TRIALS-A   (800) 874-2572
(Hearing impaired) (800) 243-7012

DDI Hotline (Bristol-Myers)
(800) 662-7999

Directory of National Helplines
(800) 678-2435

National HIV and AIDS Information Service Hotline—Dept. of Health and Human Services
(800) 342-AIDS (342-2437)
(800) 344-SIDA (344-7432) (Spanish access)
(800) AIDS-TTY (243-7889) (Deaf access)

National AIDS Information Clearinghouse
(800) 458-5231

National Institute of Health (NIH) Info. on AIDS Drug Studies
(800) AIDS-NIH (243-7644)

National Sexually Transmitted Diseases Hotline
(800) 227-8922

Project Inform (experimental/alternative treatment)
(800) 822-7422   CA (800) 334-7422

San Francisco AIDS Foundation Hotline (bilingual)
(800) FOR-AIDS (367-2437) or (415) 863-2437

AIDS / HIV INFECTION ORGANIZATIONS—NATIONAL
(check for local agencies or call national)

AID Atlanta
1132 W. Peachtree St., N.W., Atlanta, GA 30309-3624
(800) 551-2728 or (404) 876-9944 (national information)

AIDS Action Council
  2033 M St., N.W., Suite 802, Washington, D.C. 20036
  (202) 293-2886

American Association of Physicians for Human Rights
  P.O. Box 14366, San Francisco, CA 94114
  (415) 255-4547

American Foundation for AIDS Research
  1515 Broadway, Suite 3601, New York, NY 10036-8901
  (212) 719-0033

Associated Catholic Charities AIDS/ARC Initiative
  1438 Rhode Island Ave., N.E., Washington, D.C. 20018
  (202) 526-4100

Association of Lesbian and Gay Psychologists, APA
  1200 17th St., N.W., Washington, D.C. 20036
  (202) 955-7600

Federation of Parents and Friends of Lesbians and Gays
  Federation National Offices
  P.O. Box 27605, Washington, D.C. 20038
  (202) 638-4200

Gay Men's Health Crisis
  129 W. 20th St., New York, NY 10011
  (212) 807-6655

The Healing Alternatives Foundation
  (415) 626-2316

Hispanic AIDS Forum
  121 Avenue of the Americas, Suite 505, New York, NY 10013
  (212) 966-6336 or (212) 966-6662 (hotline)

Minority Task Force on AIDS
  92 St. Nicholas Ave., Suite 1B, New York, NY 10026
  (212) 749-2816

Mothers of AIDS Patients (MAP)
  c/o Ann Wright
  UCSD Medical Center, Social Work Dept., H-918
  225 Dickinson Ave., San Diego, CA 92103
  (619) 543-5730

National AIDS Information Clearinghouse
  P.O. Box 6003, Rockville, MD 20850
  (800) 458-5231

National Association of People with AIDS
1413 K St., N.W., Washington, D.C. 20005
(202) 898-0414

National Gay and Lesbian Task Force
1734 14th St., N.W., Washington, D.C. 20009
(202) 332-6483

National Hemophilia Foundation
Soho Bldg., 110 Greene St., Rm. 406, New York, NY 10012
(212) 219-8180

National Hospice Organization
1901 N. Moore St., Suite 901, Arlington, VA 22209
(703) 243-5933

National Jewish AIDS Project
2300 H St., N.W., Washington, DC 20037
(202) 296-3564

National Minority AIDS Council
300 I St., N.E., Washington, DC 20002
(202) 544-1076

People with AIDS Coalition
31 W. 26th St., Fifth Floor, New York, NY 10010
(212) 532-0290 or (212) 532-0568 (hotline)

San Francisco AIDS Foundation
P.O. Box 6182, San Francisco, CA 94101-6182
(415) 864-5855

Women's AIDS Network
c/o San Francisco AIDS Foundation
P.O. Box 6182, San Francisco, CA 94101-6182
(415) 864-5855, ext. 2007

PUBLICATIONS

AIDS/HIV Experimental Treatment Directory
American Foundation for AIDS Research
1515 Broadway, Suite 3601, New York, NY 10036-8901
(212) 719-0033

AIDS News
Hemophilia Council of CA & Northern CA Hemophilia Foundation
7700 Edgewater Dr., Ste. 710, Oakland, CA 94621-3017
(415) 568-NCHF (568-6243)

AIDS Treatment News
John S. James, P.O. Box 411256, San Francisco, CA 94141
(415) 255-0588

AIDS Update, Hemophilia Information Exchange
National Hemophilia Foundation c/o HANDI
Soho Bldg., 110 Greene St., Rm. 406, New York, NY 10012
(212) 219-8180

BETA (Bulletin of Experimental Treatments for AIDS)
San Francisco AIDS Foundation
P.O. Box 6182, San Francisco, CA 94101
(415) 863-AIDS (863-2437)

DAITA (Directory of Antiviral and Immunomodulatory Therapies for AIDS)
CDC AIDS Weekly, P.O. Box 83049, Birmingham, AL 35283-0409
(205) 991-6920

PI Perspective
Project Inform
347 Dolores St., Suite 301, San Francisco, CA 94110
(800) 822-7422   CA (415) 558-9051

PWA Coalition Newsline and *Surviving and Thriving with AIDS*
People with AIDS Coalition
31 W. 26th St., Fifth Floor, New York, NY 10010
(212) 532-0290

Treatment Issues (The GMHC Newsletter of Experimental AIDS Therapies)
Gay Men's Health Crisis, Dept. of Medical Info.
129 W. 20th St., New York, NY 10011
(212) 807-6655

READING LIST

Addiction/Recovery

The Augustine Fellowship, Sex and Love Addicts Anonymous. Boston, MA. Sex and Love Addicts Anonymous, Fellowship-Wide Services, Inc., 1986.

Alcoholics Anonymous, (The Big Book). New York, NY, Alcoholics Anonymous World Services, Inc., 1976.

Brunner, Carolyn. *For Concerned Others of Chemically Dependent Gays and Lesbians.* Center City, MN, Hazelden, 1987.

Carnes, Patrick. *Out of the Shadows: Understanding Sexual Addiction.* Minneapolis, MN, CompCare Publishers, 1983.

Diamond, Jed. *Sex and Love Addiction and Chemical Dependency: The Hidden Connection.* San Rafael, CA, Fifth Wave Press, 1989.

Finnegan, Dana and McNally, Emily. *Dual Identities: Counseling Chemically Dependent Gay Men and Lesbians.* Center City, MN, Hazelden, 1987.

Flynn, Dorothy. *AIDS and Chemical Dependency.* Center City, MN, Hazelden, 1987.

Gosselin, Renee, and Nice, Suzanne. *Lesbian and Gay Issues In Early Recovery.* Center City, MN, Hazelden, 1987.

HIVIES Manual: Human Immunodeficiency Virus Information Exchange and Support Group. Chicago, IL, HIVIES Group #1, 1989.

Hope & Recovery: A Twelve Step guide for healing from compulsive sexual behavior. Minneapolis, MN, CompCare Publishers, 1987.

Pohl, Mel and Ryan, Caitlin. *AIDS Protocol: AIDS Education and Risk-Reduction Counseling in Chemical Dependency Treatment Settings.* Rockville, MD, ARC Research Foundation, 1990.

Schaef, Anne Wilson. *Escape from Intimacy: Untangling the "Love" Addictions: Sex, Romance, Relationships.* San Francisco, CA, Harper & Row, 1989.

Tilleraas, Perry. *Circle Of Hope: Our Stories of AIDS, Addiction & Recovery.* Center City, MN, Hazelden, 1990.

Tilleraas, Perry. *The Color Of Light: Daily Meditations For All Of Us Living With AIDS.* Center City, MN, Hazelden, 1988.

The Homosexual Alcoholic: AA's Message of Hope. Center City, MN, Hazelden, 1980.

Twelve Steps and Twelve Traditions, New York, Alcoholics Anonymous World Services, Inc., 1981.

AIDS/HIV Infection

Alyson, Sasha (editor). *You Can Do Something About AIDS.* Boston, MA, The Stop AIDS Project, 1988.

Badgley, Laurence. *Choose To Live: An AIDS Healing Companion.* San Bruno, CA, Human Energy Press, 1987.

Darril, Rayna. *AIDS: The Great Awakening.* Montrose, CO, Great Awakening Press, 1988.

Hay, Louise. *The AIDS Book: Creating a Positive Approach.* Santa Monica, CA, Hay House, 1988.

Kubler-Ross, Elisabeth, *AIDS: The Ultimate Challenge.* New York, NY, Collier Books, 1987.

Melton, George. *Beyond AIDS: A Journey Into Healing.* Beverly Hills, CA, Brotherhood Press, 1988.

Nungesser, Lon. *Epidemic of Courage: Facing AIDS in America.* New York, NY, St. Martin's Press, 1986.

Pohl, Mel, Kay, Deniston and Toft, Doug. *The Caregivers' Journey: When You Love Someone with AIDS.* Center City, MN, Hazelden, 1990.

Reed, Paul. *Serenity: Support and Guidance for People with HIV.* Berkeley, CA, Celestial Arts, 1990.

Serinus, Jason (editor). *Psychoimmunity & The Healing Process: A Holistic Approach To Immunity & AIDS.* Berkeley, CA, Celestial Arts, 1986.

Shilts, Randy. *And The Band Played On: Politics, People and the AIDS Epidemic.* New York, St. Martin's Press, 1987.

Codependency/Childhood Abuse

Berry, Carmen. *When Helping You Is Hurting Me: Escaping the Messiah Trap.* San Francisco, CA, Harper & Row, 1989.

Bradshaw, John. *Healing The Shame That Binds You.* Deerfield Beach, FL, Health Communications, Inc., 1988.

Bradshaw, John. *Homecoming: Reclaiming and Championing Your Inner Child.* New York, NY, Bantam, 1990.

Forward, Susan. *Betrayal of Innocence: Incest and Its Devastation.* New York, NY, Penguin Books, 1979.

Forward, Susan. *Toxic Parents: Overcoming Their Hurtful Legacy and Reclaiming Your Life.* New York, NY, Bantam, 1989.

Kennedy, Jan. *Touch of Silence: A Healing From the Heart.* San Diego, CA, Cosmoenergetics Publications, 1989.

Kritsberg, Wayne. *The Adult Children of Alcoholics Syndrome: From Discovery to Recovery.* Deerfield Beach, FL, Health Communications, Inc., 1986.

Mellody, Pia. *Facing Codependence: What It Is, Where It Comes From, How It Sabotages Our Lives.* San Francisco, CA, Harper & Row, 1989.

Mellody, Pia. *Breaking Free: A Recovery Workbook for Facing Codependence.* San Francisco, CA, Harper & Row, 1989.

Norwood, Robin. *Women Who Love Too Much: When You Keep Wishing and Hoping He'll Change.* New York, NY, Pocket Books, 1986.

Ratner, Ellen. *The Other Side Of The Family: A Book for Recovery From Abuse, Incest and Neglect.* Deerfield Beach, FL, Health Communications, Inc., 1990.

Mind/Body

Benson, Herbert. *Beyond the Relaxation Response.* New York, NY, Berkley Books, 1985.

Borysenko, Joan. *Minding the Body, Mending the Mind.* Reading, MA, Addison-Wesley Co., 1987.

Chopra, Deepak. *Quantum Healing: Exploring the Frontiers of Mind/ Body Medicine.* New York, NY, Bantam, 1990.

Cousins, Norman. *Head First: The Biology of Hope.* New York, NY, Dutton, 1989.

Kabat-Zinn, Jon. *Full Catastrophe Living: Using the Wisdom of Your Body and Mind to Face Stress, Pain, and Illness.* New York, NY, Delacorte Press, 1990.

Locke, Steven. *The Healer Within: The New Medicine of Mind and Body.* New York, NY, Dutton, 1986.

Miller, Emmett. *Opening Your Inner "I".* Berkeley, CA, Celestial Arts, 1987.

Ornstein, Robert and Sobel, David. *The Healing Brain: Breakthrough Discoveries About How the Brain Keeps Us Healthy.* New York, NY, Simon and Schuster, 1987.

Siegel, Bernie. *Love, Medicine & Miracles: Lessons Learned About Self-Healing From a Surgeon's Experience with Exceptional Patients.* New York, NY, Harper & Row, 1986.

Siegel, Bernie. *Peace, Love & Healing: Bodymind Communication & The Path To Self-Healing—An Exploration.* New York, NY, Harper & Row, 1989.

Other

Frankl, Viktor. *Man's Search for Meaning,* New York, NY, Washington Square Press, 1963.

Keyes, Ken. *The Power of Unconditional Love: 21 Guidelines for Beginning, Improving and Changing Your Most Meaningful Relationships.* Coos Bay, OR, Love Line Books, 1990.

Jampolsky, Gerald. *Love Is Letting Go of Fear.* Berkeley, CA, Celestial Arts, 1990.

Murphy, Joseph. *The Power of Your Subconscious Mind.* Englewood Cliffs, NJ, Prentice-Hall, 1963.

IMAGERY APPENDIX

These scripts are provided so that you can make your own relaxation and affirmation tapes. In the beginning it is much easier to learn to relax and keep your mind focused if you use audio tapes as a guide. After some practice you will be able to relax anywhere, anytime without the assistance of prepared tapes. If you do the relaxation exercises that use these scripts and are suggested throughout the book you will find the other processes and steps much easier. You will also find your level of comfort and depth of feelings much deeper and more healing.

Slowly read these scripts into a tape recorder, pausing at all commas and periods. Instructions are in parentheses and are the only words that should not be read. Background music that you find comforting is very helpful. We also suggest you make a tape of the affirmations appearing throughout and at the end of each chapter. You can play these anytime during the course of your day, even when driving or working. The following relaxation exercises however, bring on deep relaxation and should not be listened to when driving or working. For the most benefit you will want to do a relaxation exercise at least twice a day and listen to your affirmation tape frequently.

For your convenience we have already made a set of tapes with Dr. Miller's soothing voice on background music. If you want to purchase rather than make your own tapes call 1-800-52-TAPES and ask for the "Living in Hope" cassettes or send in the coupon at the end of the book.

The Loving Light

This is the most basic imagery exercise. It will serve to relax and center you, mentally, physically and emotionally. You will, after a bit of practice, be able to repeat the steps from memory. They can then be used to relax deeply any time you need it, or to quickly calm yourself (through the brief technique of allowing the light to flow through and over your body). Begin each imagery exercise by reading Part 1 of this exercise and then go on to read the body of subsequent scripts.

Part 1: Deep Relaxation Script

Begin by letting yourself become aware of the fact that at this moment in time there is no place you have to go, nothing you have to do and no problem you have to solve. Take a few moments to do this.

Next, take some nice, deep breaths, slow and easy. Each time you breathe out, count ... starting with the number 1, until you've breathed twenty slow deep breaths, letting each breath out relax you even more deeply.

Now imagine that beneath your feet there is a globe of light ... a round glowing sphere of warm, healing, crystal pure light. Imagine the light as any color you choose. Maybe white or golden, or perhaps green or blue. It's your light and you can choose whatever color you want ... And as you breathe, imagine that your feet are hollow and that the soles of your feet allow light to flow in. Feel it flowing gently into your feet, into each toe as you count and breathe. With each intake of breath you are gently drawing warm, soothing light up through your feet, filling your ankles and your calves with light. Imagine them glowing from within.

Follow that light with each breath as it moves up filling your knees and your thighs, slowly ... flowing into and filling your pelvis, your buttocks, your genitals ... flowing into your abdomen and into all your internal organs. And as the light fills you, it brings relaxation ... and peace ... and a deep feeling of love.

Each rising and falling of your abdomen is like a gentle relaxation massage ... letting that pure light of relaxation flow into all the muscles of your back ... your lower back ... your upper back ... your chest ... spilling over into your shoulders ... glowing with light ... the light flowing down through your upper arms ... through your elbows and your forearms ... Comforting, soothing light flowing down through your wrists into your hands ... down into each of your fingers. Your entire body is filled with light ... from your feet all the way up to your shoulders ... peaceful, healing light flowing up into your neck, soothing and relaxing all muscles there ... filling your face ... your head ... and your scalp ... all the way to the top of your head ... Good ...

And as that warmly glowing, sphere of pure, loving energy beneath your feet continues to fill you, the light begins to overflow like a fountain out of the top of your head ... flowing out over your scalp and your head ... a shower of light flowing down over your forehead ... relaxing your forehead ... soft healing ... flowing over the muscles of your face, relaxing your jaw muscles ... relaxing ... surrounding your head and face with a soft protective glow ... like a gentle soothing protective cocoon of light spinning down around your body ... as you continue to breathe ... slowly flowing down over your neck and over your arms ...

flowing down over your fingers until it drips off your fingertips . . . making little splashes of light where it falls to the ground.

And now, not only are you filled with this healing light . . . the soft, gentle light showers you all over, from head to toe . . . bathing you in its soft protective glow . . . like standing beneath a waterfall of relaxation flowing from the top of your head, all the way over the surface of your body. Feeling the light flow down over your head and face . . . down over your neck and shoulders . . . flowing down over your chest and back . . . feel the touch of the light, the texture, the warmth . . . feeling it with all your senses . . . as it continues to flow down, surrounding your entire body, chest, abdomen, pelvis, genitals, thighs, knees, calves, ankles and feet . . . with a warm, protective, healing glow. Take a few moments to enjoy this feeling.

And now . . . filled with . . . and covered by sweet healing light, you are protected as if within a safe cocoon or crystal bubble of light. The outside of this cocoon of light is polished smooth like a mirror and it will deflect all negative energy away from you. No negative energy can enter. Inside it reflects all the positive healing energy back to you, soothing you and nurturing you . . . just let yourself stay with this wonderful, soft, soothing feeling for awhile . . . knowing that at any time during the day or night . . . anywhere you might be . . . you know you can take a deep breath in and bring this relaxed feeling back by just imagining the globe of light beneath your feet . . . And that as you breathe you breathe in that soft healing light . . . it is always there for you . . . it will always come to heal you whenever you call for it . . . this is your very own light, just breathe deeply and there it will be . . . and knowing this you rest peacefully . . .

And anytime unnecessary thoughts enter your mind, simply let the light flow into that part of your mind . . . filling the shadows with light, and washing away the thought . . . letting the thought be carried away in the stream of light flowing out . . . like a shower of shimmering diamond light flowing over your body . . . leaving you peaceful, relaxed and calm.

And now imagine that you are a *being* of light . . . and that at your center you can sense . . . at the center of all your awareness . . . a source . . . a presence . . . a spirit . . . a being . . . a voice in the silence . . . a presence beyond naming . . . that you might refer to as God or Love . . . or Universal Wisdom . . . or Life Force *(You may simply insert the one word or phrase here which best reflects the nature of your Higher Power)* . . . a Higher Power that can bring you healing and wholeness and peace.

Part 2: Loving Light Script

And imagine as the air continues to breathe for you that you can guide this healing force into your being ... by opening yourself to it, by removing all obstacles so it can do its work ... naturally, easily, lovingly.

First allowing it to flow into your mind ... bringing with it clear thinking ... accurate memory ... positive thoughts ... repeating silently within ... *(Leave about 4–10 seconds between each affirmation to give yourself time to repeat them when you listen to the tape.)*

• Today I solve problems effectively.
• Today I can deal with and grow from anger ... sadness ... and even fear and depression.
• Today I am capable of acting and thinking in new ways.
• Today my mood is stable and generally positive.
• Today I can concentrate, focus and follow through on my thoughts.

And as the soft light gently washes away all doubts, all negative thinking ... guide it into your emotions, into your feelings ... Allow the healing light into your feelings and emotions ... *(Leave about 4–10 seconds after each affirmation.)*

• Today I recognize that my feelings are only feelings ... They are neither good nor bad ... they just are.
• Today I can choose not to act on my feelings ... I no longer fear them.
• Today I can feel my feelings ... they are a part of me, and they will not harm me.
• Today I can work through my feelings and learn from them ... I don't have to avoid them.
• Today I can be with my feelings for I have an inner and outer source of strength.

Within there is a bottomless well, a limitless source of hope and energy. And with each breath, let that gentle light of relaxation, love and healing flow into every part of your body ... *(Leave about 4–10 seconds after each affirmation.)*

• I open my heart and let the healing light flow into my heart, and today I feel it being healed.
• I open my back, and chest and breathe the healing into every cell of my body.
• I open my legs and feet to the healing light, and feel them growing stronger.
• I open my arms and hands to the healing light, and feel them growing stronger and more vital.
• I open my pelvis, genitals, and abdomen to the healing light and feel its warmth working within me.

284

- I open my neck, head and face to the healing light, and feel all tensions melting away.
- With each breath my body is growing stronger.
- Today I now know how to relax myself whenever I need to, and I choose to relax often.

Now, bring to mind an image of the most relaxing, comfortable and healing place you can think of . . . a place far away from anything that could disturb you, where you could let yourself be totally at peace . . . It might be someplace you have been in the past, or it may be a place you've always wanted to go, or it could simply be an imaginary place . . .

Now imagine yourself drifting through space and time, as though you are riding on a magic carpet to this special place you have chosen . . . And as you arrive, let yourself begin to picture the sights around you there, in full color, see the movement around you . . . bring it in clearly. Imagine you can hear the sounds around you in this special place, and smell the smells, and feel the temperature . . . Bring in all the details you can . . . really let yourself be there.

And as you drift into this most wonderful place, imagine your body is as healthy and as well as you can imagine it being . . . your muscles are strong, your mind is clear, your emotions are balanced, and you feel very whole. How wonderful it feels! (*Allow 20 seconds or longer to really feel this.*)

Part 3: Reawakening

You are now the person you really want to be . . . for this is the person you already are down deep inside . . . And each time you let yourself enjoy this wonderful place you are giving your body and mind instructions to let go of all that you need to so that this naturally healthy you can express itself more freely each day of your life.

And now, as I count from one to five, let yourself gradually reorient to the physical location of your body, and return to a wide awake awareness of the space around you, coming back feeling rested, energized, and healed . . . or, if you wish, as I count you can simply let yourself continue to rest, or even drift off into a deep rejuvenating sleep.

1 . . . coming up . . . 2 . . . more and more awake . . . 3 . . . feeling refreshed and clear . . . 4 . . . bringing the relaxation with you as you become completely wide awake, opening your eyes and letting your body begin to move around, perhaps stretching and yawning . . . 5 . . . wide awake. Take a moment and notice how comfortable you feel.

Spiritual Attunement Imagery

The following imagery process helps you experience your Higher Power and allows it to help create balance and wholeness in your body, emotions, and mind.

Part 1: *Deep Relaxation* (from the Loving Light imagery, Part 1, page 282)

Part 2: *Tuning to the Spirit*

Take a deep breath in . . . and as you let it out allow your mind to clear itself of all thoughts, images and words. As the air leaves you, imagine yourself floating as though within a bubble of crystal light . . . floating higher and higher . . . lighter and lighter . . .

And at the same time, deeper within youself . . . deeper than your body . . . deeper than your emotions that come and go like rainy days and sunny days . . . deeper than the babbling brook of your thoughts that tumble and splash around the little rocks flowing through fields and meadows on its way to the sea . . . floating deeper, still deeper . . . to that place within you that has been here for a very long time . . . even before your memories . . . to the very essence of your being . . . to an immense open space of peace . . . harmony . . . and oneness.

And here in the center of the silence . . . floating silently in the stillness . . . a Presence . . . a Spirit . . . a Being . . . a Whisper in the silence . . . a Light in the darkness . . . a Presence beyond naming that you might refer to as God or Love . . . or Universal Wisdom . . . or perhaps the Life Force. A crystal clear awareness of its radiance . . . the unseen yet enormously powerful energy of your Higher Power collecting energy and swirling it about . . . creating, just as it created the very first life in the universe . . . slowly creating an energy as you move forward through time . . . through the days, weeks, or even months and years . . . envisioning an image of yourself developing . . . healing . . . gaining more and more wisdom . . . becoming more whole . . . drifting as far ahead into the future as you would like to now . . . Seeing yourself in your imagination . . . as the being you have allowed yourself to become.

And if you picture yourself in physical form, see that body as healthy . . . whole . . . comfortable . . . vigorous and energetic. You may see yourself doing anything you'd really like to be doing . . . seeing yourself as you'd really like to be . . . spiritually awake . . . aware . . . filled with love, compassion, understanding and wisdom . . . just the way you really want to be . . . *(Allow a pause of about 20 seconds.)*

And become this being and experience yourself as you and your Higher Power have created yourself. This is who you truly are . . . *(Allow a pause of about 20 seconds.)*

And as each breath breathes in, it breathes in pure light. Energy flows from this image into your physical body . . . nurturing it and transforming it into this image. And with each breath out you may repeat each of the following statements which is true . . . or you would like to become true for you. You may change any words as you wish to make it even *more* true for you as this special being . . . you and your Higher Power have created . . . yourself . . . *(Allow a pause of about 10 seconds after each affirmation.)*

- I am not my body.
- I am not my mind.
- I am not my emotions.
- I see beyond the world of the senses.
- This moment is the only moment there is.
- Only my body exists in time.
- I realize all that is physical will pass away.
- I am not attached to the physical world.
- I am guided by an inner experience of light, peace, joy and love.
- My spirit is a light that dispels darkness and fear.
- I have learned the freedom that comes with forgiveness.
- I guide all forces internal and external towards their greatest good.
- I allow love to flow through me.
- Through spirit my Higher Power and I heal my mind, my body and my spirit.

And now, if you wish you can continue to let yourself drift deeper within, to prolong this state of peace, tranquility and healing for as long as you wish, simply by turning the tape off at this moment . . . or . . . if you wish . . . you can let yourself drift back once again to that point in space and time that we call here and now . . . where your body rests . . . breathing . . . your chest and abdomen gently rising and falling with each breath . . . nurturing you . . . healing you . . . filling you with energy . . . as you gently begin to be aware of your ears, the position of your body . . . to locate your fingers and your toes . . . letting them gently begin to move as you breathe a little more deeply . . . breathing energy and wakefulness throughout your body . . . a tingling feeling . . . wanting to stretch . . . to move . . . drifting upward and becoming more and more awake . . . coming up lighter and lighter . . . feeling yourself nourished ... enriched ... inspired ... and enlightened ... by your inner experience.

Part 3: Reawakening

Gently reorienting yourself to the physical world around you ... moving your arms and legs ... And when you are ready, letting your eyelids gently open ... slowly ... allowing for the pleasant experience of the colors and shapes around you ... the sounds ... and sights ... and movement around you ... and as I count from 1 to 5 letting yourself wake up completely ... 1 ... feeling alert and refreshed ... 2 ... rested ... 3 ... as if you've been asleep for awhile ... 4 ... completely wide awake ... 5 ... now notice how comfortable you feel ...

(Use this imagery process frequently, at *least* once a day. Be patient. Soon you will begin to feel your Higher Power working daily in your life.)

Self-Healing Imagery

This imagery is to help you actually imagine yourself healing. It teaches you how to direct your inner healing light to support the healthy function of your body and immune system. It imagines your body dealing effectively with intrusions or infection and harmonizing the various organs and systems in your body.

Part 1: Deep Relaxation (from the Loving Light imagery, Part 1, page 282)

Part 2: Healing Your Body and Its Immune System

Now that you are completely relaxed and your awareness is focused within ... visualize your immune system as you imagine it to be. Your image may be symbolic, realistic or fantasy-like. The image you have is the *right* image ... it is the one *your* body will understand. Imagine all the cells of your immune system ... a vast army or team of brother and sister cells ... every one dedicated to doing its part for the highest good of the whole ... T cells, B cells, natural killer cells, macrophages, lymphocytes ... Whether or not you know them by name is not important ... however they appear to you is fine ... picture them all ... all surrounded by love and light. Imagine more and more light flowing toward them ...

as if you have a spotlight or a hose . . . or a paint brush that the light flows out of, surrounding and flowing into your many cells whose job it is to protect and heal you, just as the loving light flowed into and around you.

And now picture your T4 helper cells . . . strong . . . quick . . . capable . . . alert. Their function is to recognize all potentially harmful bacteria, viruses and other cells. Imagine that these helpful cells are very effective in identifying everything that doesn't belong in a healthy body, including infectious agents and deformed, damaged or diseased cells . . . picture your helper cells leading those unwanted visitors to the exit door and giving them a choice. They may either sleep quietly here or they must leave. Either they stay in harmony or else they have to go. Picture your immune cells ejecting any cells which have become hostile. *(PAUSE.)*

Now imagine you can stand back and watch the millions upon millions of helpful cells in your immune system at work. Imagine they are all surrounded by glowing light . . . going about their jobs perfectly. Now picture any unwanted cells, that might be the HIV virus or any other unwanted virus, bacteria or fungus you would like to be rid of. You may see them as little gray dots, or use any other image that works for you. Whatever image you use, however, make sure that you see the unwanted cells as they truly are . . . weak, confused, tired and unable to multiply. The cells are peaceful . . . non-aggressive . . .

Imagine your awareness itself is like a beam of brilliant light. Imagine that beam is growing more and more focused . . . gradually changing from a floodlight down to a razor thin laser beam. Imagine the beam of your consciousness growing smaller and more focused . . . almost as though the alert, aware part of you is shrinking down smaller and smaller. The focus of your consciousness has become like a tiny glowing dot . . . and your awareness is in that dot, suspended in front of you.

Let yourself shrink down and float across through the air into that tiny glowing point of pure loving light. Imagine that you are now suspended in the air just a few inches in front of your body. For a few moments watch your body rise and fall with each breath in . . . and out.

Now instruct your body to take a deep breath of air in . . . and as it does it breathes in this tiny point of loving light. Feel yourself being breathed into your body with this breath in . . . Visualize your air passages from the *inside* as you travel through them . . . passing across the glistening smooth membrane of your lungs into your own blood stream . . . You are now traveling through the inside of your own body, as if you are in a little submarine . . . And if you wish you can imagine you are in a tiny submarine, that can take you wherever in your body you want to go. Your purpose in being here is to invigorate and stimulate your immune system to do its job even better. Your immune system has eliminated, or put to sleep, thousands of different viruses and bacteria during your life. The task now is to repeat a performance it knows quite well.

So, whenever you encounter any unwanted virus, bacteria or fungus that is not already surrounded by soft, loving light, imagine yourself shining a beam of sparkling light on to it. If you wish you may imagine your submarine has a headlight that you can aim. Imagine the cell becoming wrapped in this light and that as this happens it becomes very drowsy ... and very sleepy ... it becomes dormant. Surrounded by love, by peace, by the loving light ... and the spirit of forgiveness and self acceptance.

Your Higher Power flows through you and surrounds it in a soft glow of tranquility and serenity ... and the cell feels safe ... and sleepy and slips into hibernation ... becoming totally dormant. As this happens all other organs and systems in your body become more peaceful, more harmonious and more perfectly balanced. The cell does not want to harm your body since this would be the end for it also. Surrounded by the loving light, all feelings of hostility within the cell are gone. It does not multiply or reproduce because it is not defensive ... nor is it hostile.

Now it's time to travel throughout your body to remind each part of your body of the healthy way it can function ... And as you travel in this little point of light, if you see anything that is amiss you will know exactly what needs to be done to correct it ... and that you have exactly the tools that you need to make that correction. Most of the time your visualizing the correct behavior is enough to restore balance.

Travel through your body to the inside of your brain. Picture the healing light as it illuminates any parts of your mind that need light. The shadows disappear as the light bathes your brain in healing, loving light ... See all the nerve cells of your body communicating to each other in a joyous and harmonious way ... Much like a symphony ... In a natural ... melodious way. Only light and love ... peace and calmness exist within your brain ... All is calm and gently quiet ... Your mind is comfortable and relaxed.

Now picture your lungs ... Imagine the air as it enters, travels around and down into the lungs. Visualize the air like pure light which expands all the little air sacs in the lungs ... The oxygen flows smoothly across the thin membrane and is easily absorbed by the blood which turns bright red as it leaves bringing oxygen to nurture the cells of the body.

See the tiny fingers which protrude from the cells that line your air passageways ... They strain any particles out of the air as they enter ...

Impurities are trapped by protective mucous which is then brought up so that your body can cough it out, thus cleansing your body . . . Your lungs are pink and well oxygenated . . . and you are coughing less and less as your lungs are more and more purified. There is an infinite supply of air around you and it enters easily. You are strong and able to exercise. There is a perfect exchange of love and light with the exchange of each breath . . . perfect harmony . . . perfect balance.

And now let your awareness travel to your skin . . . the largest organ in your body. Your skin is a protective barrier . . . an eliminator of toxins . . . a regulator of heat and cold. Your skin is clear, of normal color . . . Moisture and dryness are balanced . . . you perspire just enough to keep your body healthy . . . and no more.

And now travel down through your digestive system. Picture your throat, your stomach, and the coils of intestines within your abdomen . . . Your throat and all the mucous membranes of your body are supple, moist, free and clear . . . You have an excellent appetite and can digest all foods well . . . You absorb water well and along with it the vitamins, proteins, carbohydrates, fats, minerals, and calories that you need. These nutrients are assimilated by your body and put to good use.

Your stomach, intestine and bowel function normally. Food and water remain in them long enough to fully digest and absorb all the nutrients. Bacteria and other parasites in the intestine become weak and confused and rapidly find their way out in your well formed bowel movements . . . They do not reproduce while in the body, do not want to harm your body and do not disturb the health of your body. Any that remain in your body stay dormant.

And now with this laser thin focused beam of your consciousness . . . imagine you can look into the future, and that future you choose to look at is a positive future. You have done what you needed to do in order to bring total healing to your body, your mind, your emotions and your spirit. Travel into this positive future, and imagine looking at your body in a mirror . . . It looks healthy and strong . . . Your weight is normal . . . you have an excellent appetite, strong muscles and you are full of energy . . . Your vision is clear, bright and well focused.

You look capable of doing anything you want. Look at the muscles of your body . . . the glow of your skin . . . the sparkle of your eyes . . . the look of wisdom on your forehead . . . the look of joy and peace around your mouth. It is clear that the consciousness that inhabits this body listens to this body. This body rests when it is appropriate, exercises when it is appropriate and takes restfully energizing sleep.

Deep within you feel a sense of awe that this magnificent creation has been entrusted to you and you honor it by giving it what it needs. You listen to it and are sensitive to its requests. You have long ago ceased abusing it in any way just as you no longer abuse its thoughts, its emotions or its spirit. There is something about this body that says "I have discovered peace." *(Leave 4–10 seconds for you to repeat the affirmations.)*

- I have discovered joy.
- I have discovered my Higher Power . . . and I have surrendered my unnecessary burdens.
- Through conscious choice, dedication, and hard work I have cleared myself of all obstacles to total healing, health, wholeness and serenity.
- Deep within I have the serenity to accept those things I cannot change, the courage to change the things I can, and the wisdom to know the difference.
- I am whole, balanced, true to myself, and a reflection of the pure light of Spirit within me.

Part 3: Reawakening

You are now the person you really want to be . . . for this is the person you already are down deep inside . . . And each time you let yourself enjoy this wonderful place you are giving your body and mind instructions to let go of all that you need to so that this naturally healthy you can express itself more freely each day of your life.

And now, as I count from one to five, let yourself gradually reorient to the physical location of your body, and return to a wide awake awareness of the space around you, coming back feeling rested, energized, and healed . . . or, if you wish, you can simply let yourself continue to rest, or even to drift off into a deep rejuvenating sleep.

1 . . . coming up . . . 2 . . . 3 . . . feeling refreshed and clear . . . 4 . . . bringing the relaxation with you as you become completely wide awake . . . 5 . . . wide awake! Take a moment and notice how comfortable you feel.

Imagery for Letting Go

The following experience will provide a way for the deeper levels of your mind to release behaviors, feelings, people, thoughts, and beliefs that no longer serve to enrich your life. Many cultures provide specific rituals for times of passage, letting go of one phase of life and moving into another. The deeper levels of the mind are then much better able to move into the new phase. The following imagery can serve as your own personal ritual. Its design is partly based on time tested rituals from many cultures.

Part 1: Deep Relaxation (from Loving Light imagery, Part 1, page 282)

Part 2: Letting Go

Your entire body is relaxed and calm . . . gently protected by the soft tender light . . . here . . . now . . . just enjoying this feeling for awhile . . . a feeling as if your body is resting in the palm of a loving hand . . . as soft and relaxed as that of an infant . . . secure . . . and peaceful . . . *(Leave a pause of about 20 seconds.)*

It feels as though you have been resting here for a long, long time . . . You feel so light . . . almost weightless . . . an easy feeling. So light it feels almost as if you are gently beginning to float upward. You are surrounded by your sparkling, crystal, bubble or cocoon of soft loving light . . . floating . . . and enjoying this feeling of floating. The glowing cocoon of loving light carefully supports and protects you.

Gradually you are lifting up and floating through space and time . . . all the while remaining relaxed and peaceful. And as you enjoy this floating feeling imagine that resting there before you is a container . . . perhaps a large box . . . or any kind of container you'd like . . . in which you will be able to place all those things that you know it is time for you to let go of. If you like, it can be a beautifully decorated chest . . . perhaps skillfully crafted of stone or fine wood . . . inlaid with ivory or silver or precious stones . . . or perhaps colorfully painted . . . Or it may be a simple wooden box, or a cardboard box, or chest, sack, trash can or bag made of a very simple material . . . *(Leave a pause of about 20 seconds.)*

Any kind of container you choose . . . it is yours, available to you and only you anytime you choose to let go of something or someone . . . it is always here for you. Picture it clearly now . . . *(Leave a pause of about 20 seconds.)*

Good. Now imagine that your container, which I'll refer to as a box, is floating right here next to you . . . or in front of you . . . and that you can take it with you as you gently begin to float back through time to collect those things from your recent or distant past which it's time to let go of . . . *(Leave a pause of about 20 seconds.)*

Gradually now, you continue to relax in your cocoon of light . . . drifting back into the past . . . a pleasant, comfortable trip. You and your box surrounded by the glow of white light are gently floating back through time . . .

And now, as you continue breathing . . . without trying . . . you'll begin to notice ideas and images beginning to come to you . . . certain things it is time to let go of . . . Things you have carried with you for some time . . . things you've picked up along the journey of life . . . things you have no further need for. You've finished dealing with them . . . completed your relationship with them . . . and you know that your healing and wholeness are best served by your letting go of them. Feel your willingness to let them go . . . right now . . . a willingness to let go . . . letting go . . . safe and protected here, floating in the palm of a loving hand knowing deep within that it is truly OK to let go now . . . filled and surrounded by healing loving light. Your Higher Power is with you . . . It's OK to just let go . . . *(Leave a pause of about 20 seconds.)*

Perhaps you are at the stage of letting go of old ways of thinking . . . or doing . . . perhaps ways of responding that you developed long ago and now have no further need for. Here . . . and *now* . . . you are more aware than ever before and you want to let go of those old ways of thinking . . . and doing . . . and responding. You are choosing to let go . . . to be different . . . to be whole . . . more honest . . . more healthy. When a negative way of thinking occurs to you, hold it in mind for a moment . . . and as you breathe out let it flow out into your box . . . letting it go . . . *(Leave a pause of about 20 seconds.)*

Or perhaps you need to release patterns in your life that no longer serve you . . . habits or behaviors that you allowed yourself to become identified with rather than with the truth of who you really are. The universe and your Higher Power acknowledge and support you in this courageous work. So now, with your next breath out, breathe them into that special box . . . letting go . . . letting go of worry . . . letting go . . . *(Leave a pause of about 20 seconds.)*

Or, you may need to let go of ways of being that no longer serve your highest good . . . ways of being that no longer serve the truth of who you really are. If so, when these thoughts and images occur . . . see them briefly in your mind's eye . . . hold them for a moment in your mind . . . and your thoughts . . . and then gently let them go . . . *(Leave a pause of about 20 seconds.)*

As these images occur to you, picture them briefly in your mind's eye as though you are searching through a drawer finding old socks and worn out clothes that you no longer need . . . picturing them in your mind for only as long as you need to identify them . . . and imagine with your next breath out breathing them into your special box . . . *(Leave a pause of about 20 seconds.)* And as the image vanishes into the box . . . it vanishes from your mind . . . and from your life . . . for good . . . *(Leave a pause of about 20 seconds.)*

Good . . . With each emptying breath out . . . breathe everything you wish to release into that special box. And as you do they vanish from your thoughts . . . your mind . . . your emotions and your spirit . . . *(Leave a pause of about 20 seconds.)*

Good . . . Or, at a later stage, you may be focusing on letting go of people . . . relationships . . . people who are no longer in your life . . . bless them and send them your love . . . and if you need to, send them your forgiveness. Perhaps letting go of people you know you would be better off without . . . breathe them into the box . . . *(Leave a pause of about 20 seconds.)*

Good . . . And as these thoughts of different people pass through your mind, be willing to let go . . . willing to let go of any old or damaged relationships that no longer serve you and your higher purpose . . . Perhaps letting go of the person, or else letting go of an old useless form that the relationship has taken. Those old ways of relating are no longer you . . . let them go . . . Breathe them into the box . . . *(Leave a pause of about 20 seconds.)*

Good . . . Perhaps there are physical problems or diseases you are ready to let go of . . . breathe them into your special box . . . *(Leave a pause of about 30 seconds.)*

Perhaps there are people who are no longer on the earth plane that you need to let go of . . . picture them . . . send them your love and any other feelings that you feel the need to send them . . . Telling them anything you need to say . . . See them hearing you . . . nodding their heads as they understand your meaning . . . as they feel your heart and thoughts go out to them . . . *(Leave a pause of about 20 seconds.)* And breathe them into the loving container, surrounded by soft, gentle love and light . . . letting go with love and tenderness . . . letting go and yet knowing that you will never forget them . . . never forget the good and loving times . . . and know that those good and loving times stay with them also . . . nurturing them and nurturing you . . . but letting go of any attachments that hinder you or them evolving into the most loving place possible . . . loving here or loving in eternity . . . soft, gentle, free, and safe . . . *(Leave a pause of about 20 seconds.)*

You'll find that this box is infinitely expandable . . . it can hold everything. There is no person . . . no place . . . no thing . . . no image or idea that is too large to fit into your special container . . . when you are truly ready to let go of it. If there is anything very large that you wish to put in the container simply picture it growing smaller until it is small enough, and then breathe it out . . . watch as it floats away and slips easily and securely into your special container . . . letting go of all those things you are ready to release . . . *(Leave a pause of about 20 seconds.)*

And now visualize closing the lid on your special container and fastening it securely . . . in any way that you wish . . . you may use nails . . . glue . . . or tie it up with strong rope . . . so that you know it is securely closed . . . *(Leave a pause of about 10 seconds.)*

Let yourself stand in front of your box, your container . . . and meditate for a few moments. And in your contemplation, you are aware of how wise and valuable it will be for you to set yourself free forever from the contents of this container . . . And if you like you can surround it with flowers, perhaps picturing it in a grove of trees or some other very beautiful place of your own choosing. For you know that some of the things it contains are things that were once important to you . . . invaluable learning experiences that helped you discover your true essence . . . things that were stepping stones leading you to this moment . . . here . . . now . . . honoring them this last brief moment before letting them go . . . *(Leave a pause of about 20 seconds.)*

You might even feel a touch of sadness at this letting go . . . for sadness is a part of the cleansing process . . . of fully releasing. Yet you know that in order to grow . . . to be more free . . . to become more of who you really are . . . it is time to let go . . .

You know that if you were to open the lid and look inside you might see a replica of yourself as you have been in the past. In many ways what is in the box is like you were . . . it has characteristics that you had . . . In many ways it might seem to be you . . . yet deep within you know it is *not* the *real* you . . . it is not your essence . . . it is not your authentic higher self. For you can feel *whole* without these things . . . feel your true nature within yourself now . . . relieved of the burden the past may have held for you.

And if you'd like . . . before finally releasing the box and all that is within it, you may wish to bid them goodbye or have a ceremony of some kind. Perhaps a solemn ceremony . . . or a celebration with music and balloons and streamers . . . a celebration for the rebirth of your true nature . . . a party of the first order . . . whatever *you* choose . . .

And you may do this alone . . . with loved ones . . . or a teacher . . . or as many people as you wish in this scene . . . now . . . *(Leave a pause of about 20 seconds.)*

Now it is time to take leave of this box, with all of your reflections and memories of you as you have been in the past . . . If you wish you may take a moment and surround it with white light . . . white light flowing from within you . . . from the source within you . . . flowing out and surrounding the container with a white glow . . . Take a deep breath in and picture your container beginning to float away from you . . . pushing it away if you wish . . . releasing it into the swiftly moving river of time . . . Watch it as it leaves . . . moving away from you, slowly at first, then faster and faster as the current begins to take it . . . it is safe to let it go.

And as it becomes more distant it starts to look smaller and smaller, as distant things do . . . And as it becomes smaller and smaller it is beginning to glow brighter and brighter, as if on fire in the distance . . . and in the distance where it appears very tiny you can see the pure white light radiating from it as if it were a star or a small sun or planet . . . Feel the warmth of that light as it reaches you and flows over you warming you as you might be warmed by the sun . . . *(Leave a pause of about 10 seconds.)*

It has become one of myriad other points of light in the distance. And the light from all these points of light shines down upon you and the space around you and upon the entire planet. And imagine that these points represent guides . . . teachers . . . some that you have experienced in the past . . . perhaps some that you have yet to meet as you continue on your journey . . . feeling the light showering down from all these glowing points . . . flowing down and enveloping the earth in a luminous . . . iridescent . . . shimmering chrysalis of white light, of loving energy, of peace. Feeling yourself at the center of this chrysalis . . . this cocoon . . . and sensing within that quiet knowing . . . a oneness . . . of peace . . . sustained by the loving energy around you . . . *(Leave a pause of about 20 seconds.)*

And focus now upon this essence . . . upon the essence of your awareness . . . this quiet center . . . imagining it like a seed planted at the very center of your being. Experience the light from above surrounding this seed, and the seed, surrounded by light . . . growing warmer . . . Feel the love . . . the softness and warmth from your heart flowing out gently like rain . . . watering the seed. And imagine it germinating now, beginning to send out roots . . . roots growing downward . . . downward toward the earth . . . flowing downward through your pelvis . . . genitals and thighs . . . down through your knees and legs and feet . . . through your toes and the soles of your feet . . . strong vigorous roots growing out from this seed . . . deep into the earth . . . *(Pause for about 20 seconds.)*

And as the light from above continues to bathe the seed . . . a stem . . . reaches upward . . . a soft . . . tender . . . green . . . stem . . . stretching upward . . . with branches . . . and leaves . . . spreading to receive the light

... reaching up ... stretching up ... climbing up ... sending branches higher and higher ... branches spreading like arms with leaves ... green leaves drinking in the light ... and blossoms of light ... soft pink ... their delicate petals fluttering down with each little breeze ... fluttering down like a fragrant snowstorm to fall softly to the earth beneath ... And nestled among the leaves and blossoms ... a most beautiful bird sings ... filling the air with sweet music ... *(Leave a pause of about 20 seconds.)*

And the melody seems to come from within you ... an inner symphony ... flowing down through you bringing a new kind of life ... Awakening movement within you ... a movement that is more free ... more joyful ... more in harmony with your Higher Power and more in harmony with your Higher Self's will for you ...

You are new ... being reborn every minute of every day. And if any time concerns or worries should come along you will remember this experience ... and as you breathe white light through your body you can choose to breathe those concerns or worries out ... to let them go ... just as you have done here ... simply by willing it to be so.

Part 3: Reawakening

And now gently ready yourself to return ... to reorient yourself to your physical body and the space around you knowing that you have your special box always available to you to use ... knowing that you can use this container anytime you wish to release any daily concerns and problems.

Gently feel yourself returning ... coming back full of enthusiasm and hope ... letting the inner music within you awaken you to the beauty of life that beckons to you ... more and more awake ... alert ... refreshed ... comfortable and clear ... 1 ... coming up ... 2 ... more and more awake ... 3 ... 4 ... completely wide awake ... 5.

And notice how comfortable you feel.

Image Rehearsal for Writing Your Own Script

This experience will provide an opportunity to increase your awareness of your emotional potential, and to become more sensitive to the range and subtlety of your feelings. It will also teach you to trust your feelings, to balance them, and to use your emotional state as an important guide in making decisions and choices in your life, especially those involving your health and wellness.

Part 1: Deep Relaxation (from Loving Light imagery, Part 1, page 282)

Part 2: Image Rehearsal

Tune into your breathing. Feel the rising and falling of your chest and abdomen with each breath. Take a deep breath in and as you let it out, imagine you're a balloon letting out all the air completely flat and relaxed . . . Just let the breathing do itself . . . Imagine the air is breathing you . . . Repeat the words in your mind, "it breathes me," and with the breathing out, let yourself feel a sense of letting go . . .

Notice that after the air leaves your body, and just before the little spark comes along that starts your next breath, there's a short pause . . . The air breathes in for you, then there's a letting go, then a little pause before the next breath begins itself . . . This is the quietest point of the breathing cycle.

Imagine with each breath out the loving light is being breathed out like a mist . . . and that this mist becomes visible, and with each breath out imagine this mist is taking a physical shape in front of you. Imagine that it forms an image of you looking and feeling the way you'd like to look and feel—looking calm and relaxed. And perhaps at first, you may only get a flash of an image or a blurry one—but gradually you begin to see and feel this image more and more clearly. See yourself looking healthy, strong, and serene; an image of yourself just the way you really want to be . . . *(Leave 10 seconds for this image to form clearly.)*

And now, with each breath in, imagine breathing this image into your self, letting it fill your body . . . Always letting the air do the breathing for you.

Now as you continue to enjoy seeing and experiencing this image and the quiet breathing, allow yourself to notice the feelings in your chest and upper abdomen . . . Just feel what you feel without attempting to name your emotions . . . Sometimes they may be calm and unruffled, like a peaceful lake. Sometimes they may be fiery, energetic, radiating strength, vitality, and power. And sometimes your emotional state may be somewhere in between. Don't attempt to change how you feel, just feel what you feel, right now . . . And accept it . . . Sometimes you may feel sadness or despair . . . And sometimes joy . . . Sometimes fear and anxiety . . . Uncertainty . . . Sometimes a loving warmth . . . And sometimes anger or resentment . . . Sometimes enthusiasm and inspiration.

Allow yourself to experience what you feel as you repeat each phrase I offer. With each breathing out repeat the phrase silently within. And if you wish, you may change any of these positive self statements slightly, so that they correspond more closely to *your* values and to the person you want to be. *(Allow 4–10 seconds as needed after each affirmation.)*

- I can allow myself to be calm. I can stay honest, open minded and willing.
- I am receptive and accepting. I can allow myself to be at peace.
- I can be patient.
- I can know serenity.
- I open myself to joy and happiness.
- I can choose to let go of attachments and to ideas. I can let go of feelings and objects without fear of loss.
- Within, I possess a limitless store of peace and love.
- My Higher Self works for my highest good.
- I have learned to calm my emotions at will.
- My Higher Power does for me that which I cannot do for myself.

Good! . . . Now take a deep breath in, and as you let it out again, let it be a feeling of letting go . . . let the air continue to breathe for you . . . Let yourself become aware now of the breathing *in* part of your cycle— aware of the inspiration . . . And, with each breathing in, repeat each of the following phrases silently within . . . *(Pause 4–10 seconds after each affirmation.)*

- I feel confidence and strength from within.
- I can assert myself and be expressive.
- I can draw upon a vast inner source of energy and power.
- I can direct this energy toward my highest good.
- My inner strength allows me to confront and experience emotions of sadness, fear, and anger.
- My Higher Power gives me the strength to successfully resist any negative influence I choose to.
- My Higher Self is powerful and capable.
- I can fight with great courage.
- I can accept with great calm.

Good! . . . And now, with each breath in, repeat internally the phrase, "I am responsible for my emotions." And as you breathe out, the phrase, "My emotions serve my mind, my body, and my spirit." . . . *(Leave a pause of about 20 seconds.)* The statements that you have made to yourself will continue to echo within.

Now it's time to practice writing your own script. To use image rehearsal to create a desirable outcome in a future situation, imagine yourself now in the kind of situation that might have been difficult for you to handle in the past; a time when you might have slipped into unhealthy behavior patterns or made choices that were not in your best long-term interest. Perhaps the kind of situation in which you might have let your emotions run away with you ... *(Leave a pause of about 20 seconds.)*

That was then, when you were using your own power. This is now and today your Higher Power is working in you to remove these character defects. Now imagine that exactly the same scene is about to take place again. But you are different now, and you will handle it differently. As you go forward into the future, set the scene clearly. See where you are, what you're doing. But this time, as you go through it, allow your Higher Power to write your script. You are sensitive to your feelings, but not a slave to them. You are able to feel angry, happy, sad, enthusiastic, fearful, loving, or any of a thousand subtle variations. The emotions you feel help you to understand the situation. You relax, focus and decide how you wish to respond, knowing the choice of how to behave is yours to make ... *(Leave a pause of about 20 seconds.)*

Feel yourself making the correct choices, with full clarity, feeling responsible to your true self, drawing on your Higher Power assertiveness. See yourself relaxed and receptive, and yet energetic and assertive. Hear your voice as you speak out of a center of calm, and act this scene through—just the way you would like to ... Sensitive ... Alert ... Clear minded ... Expressive ... Assertive ... *(Leave a pause of about 60 seconds.)*

Now let this scene fade away and bring to mind *another* situation which might actually happen in the future, a situation in which you would like to behave in a certain way. Perhaps you want to confront someone. Perhaps you would like to be calm instead of upset as you would have been in the past. Choose the kind of situation where it might, in the past, have been hard to make the healthy choice ... *(Leave a pause of about 20 seconds.)* Now, as you go through this scene, see yourself acting out of that place deep within that has all the answers—has all the strength and courage to carry you through whatever situation you choose to rehearse now. You are no longer alone. Your Higher Power works with you and through you ... *(Leave a pause of about 60 seconds.)*

Good ... You may choose to use this rehearsal for strength about new, safe sexual behavior or new assertive ways of declining drugs and alcohol, perhaps to dispel fears concerning doctor appointments or lab tests. Let yourself use this experience often, either with or without the tape. Any time you anticipate an event that presents a challenge you can mentally rehearse and empower yourself for the real event. Each time you use your imagination in this way you are reinforcing the image and outcome that you want.

Part 3: Reawakening

Now, as I count from one to five, allow yourself to come to full wakefulness feeling refreshed, alert, calm, with a pleasant feel of excitement within . . . or, if you wish, you may use the counting to guide you into a state of deep restfulness. And each time you picture yourself looking and feeling the way you want to look and feel, you become more and more the person you really want to be—the person you already are down deep inside . . . 1 . . . coming up . . . 2 . . . more and more awake . . . 3 . . . feeling your body beginning to want to move, perhaps moving your hands and feet . . . 4 . . . maybe stretching your arms or legs . . . 5 . . . taking a deep breath in, and as you let it out, letting your eyelids open—wide awake, comfortable, and notice how good you feel.

Suggestions for Using Imagery Tapes

1. Get comfortable. If you lie down, let your spine sink towards the surface you are on, perhaps supporting your knees or the small of your back with pillows. If you sit upright, keep your spine vertical so you don't put any strain on your back muscles.

2. Relax the muscles of your face, your shoulders, and your upper back. Don't be concerned about what you look like!

3. Breathe from your diaphragm, so that your lower belly, or abdomen, rises a little as you breathe in and sinks back as you exhale, as if there is a balloon inflating and deflating in your abdomen.

4. Try to listen to the tape in a quiet room that has soft lighting, where you won't be interrupted by the telephone, family, or visitors. (You can put a note on the door and leave the phone off the hook.)

5. Most people keep their eyes closed which helps with concentration. If you wear glasses, remove them.

6. You may become more relaxed than you are used to, and even feel a little out of control, but *you're not*. Just clench a fist, open your eyes or voice a sound and you'll know that you are *okay*.

7. Don't worry if you have thoughts going through your mind while you're listening. Most people do. When you recognize such a thought just let it go and gently refocus on the words on the cassette.

8. There is no one "right way" of doing this. *Exactly what you are doing is right for you at the time.* Like all skills, this one takes learning and practice. You will become more expert with time.

9. You may have some novel sensations, perhaps a feeling of light floating or of tingling in your hands. Don't worry about these experiences. Just enjoy them, and recognize that they reflect the positive inner changes that you are undergoing.

MEETING APPENDIX

How to Start a Meeting

1. Propose adding or extending an already established support group using this program, or start a new group.

2. Find a location for the meeting by asking at AIDS or other resource centers for churches, banks, and community or counseling centers that donate or inexpensively rent a room.

3. Put a notice up on bulletin boards, in local newspapers, and church, AIDS, and gay community newsletters stating type of group, time, and location. (For example: "HIV Anonymous Group, using a program based on AA Twelve Steps, Thursday 7–9 pm, Community room at United Methodist Church on Grape and Ash.")

4. Ask at centers for phone numbers of people who are known to already be in Twelve Step Programs and ask their help. (They will probably know how to start a meeting.)

5. Pick a time that doesn't conflict with other popular meetings.

6. Make a list of people to make announcements about the meeting and help distribute flyers.

7. Make a list of places to distribute or post flyers.

8. Ask a few of your friends to be there for the first few meetings.

9. If you like, photocopy the meeting format in this chapter or make your own.

It is our experience and the experience of others that unless there is some structure to the meeting it will end up being a free for all session and not last long. Those kinds of sessions may be necessary but that is not the purpose of this program.

Format

(This is adapted from formats used in AA and other Twelve Step Programs.)

Welcome

My name is _____ and I am affected by HIV. I am your leader for this meeting. We want to welcome you to the Thursday night meeting of HIV Anonymous. I'd like to begin the meeting with a few minutes of silent meditation followed by the Serenity Prayer. I would like to suggest to those of you who may be new to this program a guided imagery for meditation. Just sit comfortably with your hands resting in your lap and your legs uncrossed. For the next three minutes imagine a light coming up into your feet and slowly filling your entire body as you inhale. Then imagine the light flowing out of the top of your head and flowing down over and covering your entire body. Relax and let this image of healing light fill your entire body as well as cover and protect your entire body. *(Pause 3 minutes)* and now the Serenity Prayer.

THE SERENITY PRAYER

God, grant me the serenity to accept the things I cannot change,
The courage to change the things I can,
And the wisdom to know the difference.

(Leader) I've asked _____(name)_____ to read the Preamble.

Preamble

Hi. My name is _____ and I am affected by HIV. HIV Anonymous is an anonymous fellowship of men and women who wish to heal themselves and their relationship to themselves and others and overcome the problems related to HIV infection. We share with one another our experience, strength, and hope in the attitude of solving our common problems and helping others to recover. The only requirement for membership is having your life affected by HIV and a desire for healthy, loving, and accepting relationships with your total self and others.

HIV Anonymous is self-supporting through our own contributions. We are not allied with any sect, denomination, politics, organization, or institution. We do not wish to engage in any controversy. We neither endorse nor oppose any causes.

We rely upon the wisdom, knowledge, Twelve Steps, and Twelve Traditions, as adopted for our purpose from Alcoholics Anonymous, as the principles of our program and guides to living healthy lives. Although separate entities, we should always cooperate with all twelve-step recovery programs.

(Leader) Thank you _____.
I have asked _____ to read the Twelve Steps.

Twelve Steps of HIV Anonymous

Hi. My name is _____ and I am affected by HIV.

1. We admitted that we are powerless over being at risk or infected with the AIDS virus, that our lives had become unmanageable.

2. Came to believe that a Power greater than ourselves could restore us to sanity.

3. Made a decision to turn our wills and our lives over to the care of God as we understand God.

4. Made a searching and fearless moral inventory of ourselves.

5. Admitted to the God of our understanding, to ourselves, and to another human being the exact nature of our wrongs.

6. Became entirely ready to have the God of our understanding remove all these defects of character.

7. Humbly asked the God of our understanding to remove our shortcomings.

8. Made a list of all persons we had harmed, and became willing to make amends to them all.

9. Made direct amends to such people wherever possible, except when to do so would injure them or others.

10. Continued to take personal inventory, and when we were wrong, promptly admitted it.

11. Sought through prayer and meditation to improve our conscious contact with God, as we understand God, praying only for knowledge of God's will for us and the power to carry that out.

12. Having had a spiritual awakening as the result of these steps, we try to carry this message to other people affected by HIV, and to practice these principles in all our affairs.

(Leader) Thank you _____.

We read the Twelve Traditions on the first Thursday of the month and today I have asked _____ to read them.

Twelve Traditions of HIV Anonymous

Hi. My name is _____and I am affected by HIV.

1. Our common welfare should come first; personal recovery depends on HIV A unity.

2. For our group purpose there is but one ultimate authority—a loving Higher Power as expressed by our group conscience. Our leaders are but trusted servants; they do not govern.

3. The only requirement for membership is the desire to heal those areas of your life that are affected by HIV.

4. Each group should remain autonomous except in matters affecting other groups or HIV Anonymous as a whole.

5. Each group has but one primary purpose—to carry its message to others affected by HIV who still suffer.

6. A HIV Anonymous group ought never endorse, finance or lend the HIV Anonymous name to any related facility or outside enterprise, lest problems of money, property and prestige divert us from our primary purpose.

7. Every HIV Anonymous group ought to be fully self-supporting, declining outside contributions.

8. HIV Anonymous should remain forever nonprofessional, but our service centers may employ special workers.

9. HIV A, as such, ought never be organized; but we may create service boards or committees directly responsible to those they serve.

10. HIV A has no opinion on outside issues; hence the HIV A name ought never be drawn into public controversy.

11. Our public relations policy is based on attraction rather than promotion; we need always maintain personal anonymity at the level of press, radio, and films.

12. Anonymity is the spiritual foundation of all our traditions; ever placing principles before personalities.

Guidelines for Sharing

(Leader) The guidelines for sharing are as follows:

This is an anonymous program so you may identify yourself by your first name only.

The thoughts and feelings shared in this meeting are shared in the strictest confidence and should remain here.

To allow the person sharing to have continuity of thought there will be no cross talk or interrupting.

We refrain from advice giving. We are all welcome to share our experiences and what has worked for us, but our choices are our own; no one should advise another person on what to do. The exception to that may be newcomers seeking advice from sponsors.

We refrain from criticizing. This program fosters unconditional acceptance of ourselves and others. Feel free to ask for feedback from other members but refrain from unsolicited criticism.

Stick to the topic at hand. We are here to discuss how we live comfortably with HIV affecting our lives. We are not here to judge or discuss pros or cons on specific treatment strategies or political issues. There are other places to do that. Here we stick to the steps and principles of Twelve Step Programs.

(Leader) This meeting is a step/chapter study. We start reading with the introduction and pick up where we left off at the next meeting. The Format for this meeting is that a person reads from the book several paragraphs and then shares on what was just read. If another member of the group would also like to share on that specific piece he or she may raise their hand after the sharing so that the leader can acknowledge them. Please keep your sharing to five minutes so that everyone gets a chance to share.

This meeting is ninety minutes long. We will read from the book for the first hour and the next thirty minutes will be spent sharing on the general aspects of the readings of today or any specific concerns or problems. If for any reason you do not have a chance to share during the meeting be sure to get together with another member after the meeting. Do not leave here without connecting and sharing what you need to share. The basket is passed during the secretary's announcements, for according to the Seventh Tradition, we are self supporting, declining outside contributions.

(Leader) Can we go around the room first and introduce ourselves and then start reading with _____(name)_____ ?

... (one hour later) *(Leader)* We will stop the reading now and open the meeting for discussion. Who would like to share, remembering to keep your sharing from 3–5 minutes so more will have a chance to share?

(A step study meeting is one type of meeting. We feel that until the entire book is studied as a group that would be the best approach. But there are many other types of meetings. There are 7 A.M. Monday "attitude adjustment" breakfast meetings and Friday Nite-Live Midnight meetings. People have candlelight meetings on the beach and tailgate meetings in parking lots. After you feel comfortable you can be as creative as you want as long as you stick to the steps and traditions. There are speaker meetings as well as discussion meetings. Some topics for discussion meetings might be any of the headings in the book, like how to handle anger, or depression or guilt, safe sex or disclosure issues, etc.)

Ending the Meeting

(Leader) I'll turn the meeting over to the secretary _____.

(Secretary, who is in charge of collecting donations for and paying the rent) I'll send the basket for donations around while I make any announcements. Are there any HIV A related announcements from the group? Any non-HIV A announcements? (The secretary makes any announcements, for instance new meetings being started.)

Is there anyone who cannot get out to a meeting that we can take a meeting to or give an extra call? Anyone we need to send a card to?

Can I have a volunteer to lead next week's meeting? I'd like to thank _____ for a great meeting and turn the meeting back over to him for the final meditation.

(Leader) Can we stand in a circle for a moment of silence and send healing energy and loving thoughts to those who still suffer and then will you _____ lead us in a prayer of your choice. (Usually join hands or arms and say the Serenity Prayer or the Lord's Prayer.)

INDEX

importance of social network in,
134, 225
minimizing risk of, 234
ninth step and, 180–181
no longer death sentence, 1–2
and opportunistic infections, 235
premature death as possibility, 230
reaction to, 27, 29, 84, 145
requires many life changes, 152–153
sixth step and, 142
stages of emotional responses to, 238
substance abuse and, 247–248
tenth step helps deal with, 198–199
transmission of, 77, 234–236, 241–242
twelfth step and, 219
unique challenges of, 245–246
value of testing for, 247
HIV positive
defined, 17
high-risk sexual behavior while, 73–74
Homophobia
accepting the fact of, 187
as danger, 136
Homosexual community
stress and, 62–63
substance abuse in, 34, 248
Honesty, avoiding through denial, 23, 25
Hostility, dealing with, 186–189
Human immunodeficiency virus. *See* HIV
infection
Humility
defining, 153
developing, 125
Ideal Self. *See* Authentic Self
Imagery
effect on immune cells through, 64
spiritual attunement through, 80–82
to enhance the twelve-step program, 13
use of, 37–38, 155, 178, 251–252
Immune system
as defense system, 61–62
depression and, 64, 90–91
meditation and, 212
stress and, 62–63
thought patterns and, 65–66
Induced feelings, defined, 75
Infection, how to avoid, 2
Infection status, how to manage
uncertainty over, 2
Inner child
making amends to, 192–193
touching the wounded, 117–119
Inner-child groups, as support, 119
Inner Healer, behavior which supports,
92, 94–95

Insane behaviors
definition of, 61
drug and alcohol cofactors as, 79–80
sexual cofactors as, 78–79
which increase risk, 77
See also Sanity
Interleukin 1, effect of marijuana on, 31
Inventory
of emotions, 199–200, 202
taking life, 221
Irrational beliefs
challenging, 66
identified, 65
Irreversible thinking, as destructive, 67
IV drug usage
AIDS advance through, 19
risk of, 32–33
stress and, 62–63
James, William, on discovery of
spirituality, 220
Jung, Carl, on the eternal child, 112
Kaposi's sarcoma (KS)
defined, 63
diagnosis of, 6
Kennedy, Jan, on characteristics of
abused, 161–162
Kiecolt-Glaser, Janice, on effect of
meditation on immune system, 212
King, Martin Luther Jr., as positive
example, 223
Kobasa, Suzanne, studies on hardiness,
68–69
KS. *See* Kaposi's sarcoma
KY jelly, used in protected sex, 78
Labels, dangers of, 114
Laperriere, on benefits of exercise, 101
Latency period, of HIV infection, 246
Latent viruses, reactiviation of, 17
Legitimate rights, vs. mistaken
assumptions, 71–72
Letting go
imagery for, 130
process for, 131–132
Life review, as part of fourth step,
115–116. *See also* Self-examination
Life as unmanageable. *See*
Unmanageability
Living, reasons for, 98, 231–232
Living in Hope
audiocassettes used in imagery, 13
twelve-step program as basis of,
247–251
Long-term survivors (LTS)
characteristics of, 220–221, 226,
249–250
definition of, 7

For people with AIDS, ARC or HIV infection . . .

LIVING IN HOPE
(three audio cassettes for $24.95)

Based on this book, *Living in Hope,* this series of tapes will help you understand how the life-promoting skills of deep relaxation, guided visualization, and positive affirmation fit into a total program of caring for yourself when you have AIDS or are infected with HIV.

The experiences on these cassettes are designed to assist you at every level—mental, emotional, physical, and spiritual—in your healing effort.

Contents of the cassette series:

> **Cassette 1**
> *Side A:* Using this Program: how and why it works.
> *Side B:* The Loving Light Within: guided imagery to a peaceful place within.
>
> **Cassette 2**
> *Side C:* Tuning to Spirit: contacting the higher power within.
> *Side D:* Healing Imagery: learn to direct your inner healing light.
>
> **Cassette 3**
> *Side E:* Visualization for Letting Go: releasing the pain of the past.
> *Side F:* Image Rehearsal for a New Inner Script: use your inner power to write a new script for your future.

To order by phone, call toll-free 1-800-52-TAPES and charge to your VISA or Mastercard.

Or order by mail, sending $24.95 (plus $3.25 postage and handling in continental U.S.; $3.50 in Hawaii, Alaska, or Canada; or $10 for overseas air). Make checks and money orders (U.S. funds only) payable to SOURCE. Or charge to your VISA or Mastercard by sending your account number, expiration date, and signature. Send your order to: SOURCE, P.O. Box W, Stanford, CA 94309.